ADVANCE PRAISE

Anyone with a stake in patient care, patient experience, population health, or health system leadership will find this book to be an unparalleled and foundational tool to create meaningful and lasting progress in our industry."

—R. ALLEN COFFMAN, MD
MEDICAL DIRECTOR, PEDIATRIC HEALTHCARE
IMPROVEMENT INITIATIVE FOR TENNESSEE

David's passion for human understanding and patient-centricity is palpable and to be applauded. In this book, he elegantly aligns anthropology and design thinking to support the biopsychosocial model of care that is foundational to our healthcare system of tomorrow.

—KALEB MICHAUD, PHD
DIRECTOR OF FORWARD, THE NATIONAL DATABANK
FOR RHEUMATIC DISEASE; ASSOCIATE PROFESSOR OF
MEDICINE, UNIVERSITY OF NEBRASKA MEDICAL CENTER

As an anthropologist devoted to healthcare, I know this book will change the careers and lives of many healthcare executives. The insights you will learn are foundational and necessary for those of us seeking to do better work on behalf of patients and HCPs. Important context for the emerging generation of healthcare executives.

—MATTHEW BRADLEY
HEALTHCARE ANTHROPOLOGIST AND ETHNOGRAPHER

WHAT'S THEIR STORY?

WHAT'S THEIR STORY?

Anthropology, Design Thinking, and
The Rebirth of Healthcare Marketing

DAVID McDONALD

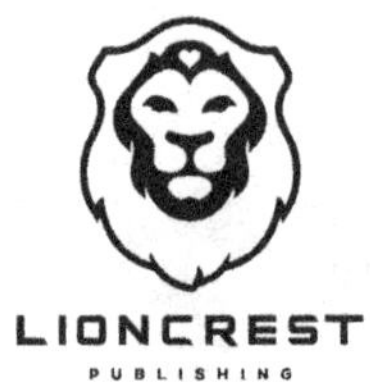

COPYRIGHT © 2020 DAVID MCDONALD

WHAT'S THEIR STORY?
Anthropology, Design Thinking,
and the Rebirth of Healthcare Marketing

ISBN   978-1-5445-1413-0 *Hardcover*
        978-1-5445-1412-3 *Paperback*
        978-1-5445-1411-6 *Ebook*

This book would not have been possible without the experience of working with so many talented professionals over the course of my career as a healthcare entrepreneur. To that end, I want to dedicate this book to my professional network—the many team members of my businesses and the many colleagues with whom I have worked and from whom I have learned much over the years. Thank you.

CONTENTS

INTRODUCTION

I've always had an empathic sensibility even before I realized it was an important characteristic for an anthropologist. If a fellow student sat alone at lunch, I joined them. If someone was bullied, I defended them. In every aspect of my life, I'm genuinely concerned about what other people think, feel, and need—it's a blessing and a curse.

My college journey began with the study of art and art history despite my curiosity in a myriad of subjects. I loved art and enjoyed history, so the combination of these interests made the most sense to me at the time. It's safe to say that I was less than settled in college, and I shape-shifted more than once as I explored the opportunities afforded to me in higher education. As my majors, minors, and emphases evolved, one thing never wavered: my passion for learning about the world around me. Thankfully, I landed on anthropology as a primary area of focus in school and it's there where a foundation was built for my career as an entrepreneur.

I confess, my love for anthropology was a happy accident. I enrolled in an anthropology class to fulfill a credit need—not knowing what anthropology was—or that the course would change my entire outlook on life. One day, a professor, Dr. Miles, gave a presentation about a research study she was leading on apes and sign language at the university. In the stories and visuals she shared, she and Chantek, an orangutan, used sign language to communicate and connect on a level that mesmerized me.

Not even twenty-four hours passed before I was in Dr. Miles' office. I wanted to learn everything I could about Chantek, and I was determined to be a part of the research study in any way possible. Dr. Miles kindly listened to my expression of interest and then asked if I knew American sign language. Surprisingly, I did. I explained to her that I had a friend who was deaf when I was a child, and I taught myself sign language as a Boy Scout so that my friend and I could communicate. Unfortunately, that wasn't enough—I needed to be fluent and certified for qualification. With no further direction or explanation, she ushered me out.

I returned a few months later with a certificate for a completed sign language course in my hand. With that single certificate, I joined the study and changed the course of my future.

It didn't take long for me to realize that I'd found my calling. I studied linguistics and language acquisition in nonhuman primates, and I learned the universal importance of gestures and body language in communication. I also explored how apes interpret the idea of currency and even how they recall locations and practice deception.

For the first time in my life, I was passionate and focused. I changed my major to anthropology, which confused my entire family who had dedicated their careers to business and journalism. My grandfather (a newspaperman) was fond of telling his friends that they could easily spot me on campus most any time of day. I was the one with a monkey on my back. "The one without the tail," he would say. Of course, I always corrected him that Chantek was an ape, not a monkey, and that apes don't have tails.

One of the most important things I learned from my days studying anthropology and my time with Chantek was the meaning and value of empathy. I discovered how it works at the most fundamental level of connection between two beings. I never truly understood empathy or its significance to me until my studies shifted to anthropology.

THE IMPACT OF EMPATHY

I first read about empathy and cultural understanding in an article discussing anthropological fieldwork. It was a rather controversial article by Clifford Geertz, which explored ethnography—the study of humans in their natural and lived environment. It caught my attention that a focus of study existed where researchers observed individual people to discern each person's reality. Through careful observation, ethnographers can study the intricacies of human social behavior, but more than that, they can achieve a better understanding of what motivates that behavior. In the article, the anthropologist discussed how leveraging observation and empathy can lead to a better understanding of the culture and community in which the person was immersed.

I was more than intrigued—I was hooked. These lessons became the basis for my understanding of the world and the people in it. Not only did I grasp the significance of empathy, but I finally understood how empathy related to the people I came in contact with.

When I left college and worked as an assistant elementary school teacher, I used what I learned about empathy and human behavior to engage with the schoolchildren on their level. As a bartender, I found myself using empathy as I served drinks and carefully listened to stories of hardship and glory. When I started True North, my first healthcare marketing agency, empathy was at the core of our company culture and business philosophy.

It was at True North that I became keenly aware of two truths central to my identity and personal mindset. The first was that no matter the industry, we as business leaders must strive to better understand and be more relevant to the needs of others in order to serve them to our fullest capacity. The second was that the people we work with carry as much importance as the clients we serve.

Now I understand that empathy is at the very core of who I am—it's at the core of everything I do in both my public and private life. Above all, empathy provides the cornerstone for the work I do in building businesses that are intent on developing patient-centered solutions in healthcare.

I care about people with both emotional and cognitive empathy, and I appreciate it when others care about me. Empathy serves a basic human need for validation and is a powerful tool for healthcare professionals interested in empowering successful outcomes—clinically or financially.

True North was a strong, successful company when I sold it. Our success was because of the human connections we shared with one another as co-workers and with the clients we were fortunate enough to work with on a daily basis. I took this approach and used it as the foundation for LIFT, a marketing and design firm focused on the healthcare space and the patients within it. I sought to leverage empathic concern in healthcare marketing—to listen to patients rather than speak to them. Empathy can break down barriers in almost every setting and circumstance, and I wanted LIFT and our clients to use it as our greatest resource.

Without my research and studies in anthropology, none of this would have been possible. Studying anthropology and design showed me how empathy could be used to understand the human condition at an unprecedented level. As a healthcare marketing strategist, I've learned how valuable empathy is in my work. Empathy *should* be used in business—but it *must* be used in healthcare.

THE EMPATHY TRIAD

In order to understand the value of empathy in healthcare, it's important to first define it. Google and Merriam-Webster will tell you that empathy is the ability to understand and share the feelings of another. To better illustrate and expand on this definition, I think empathy is best defined within the context of the empathy triad. The empathy triad is a nice way of framing and evaluating how you view empathy and your relative strength or needs in each of three areas—cognitive empathy, emotional empathy, and empathic concern.

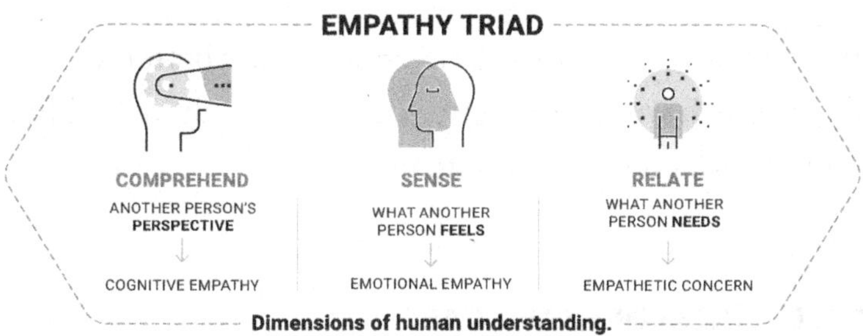

Cognitive empathy is the ability to understand another person's perspective by putting yourself in their shoes. Emotional empathy is the ability to feel what someone else is feeling. Empathic concern is the ability to sense what another person needs from you.

This gets to the heart of patient-centeredness and is the very reason we use ethnography for healthcare marketing strategy and solution design.

Providers need to recognize that there's a reason why their patients do the things they do. It's not uncommon for healthcare professionals to get frustrated with people when they fall short of expectations. Some providers may even give up on difficult patients or stakeholders. Because of this, patients *and caregivers* can often get lost in the system. This is an unnecessary outcome and one that can be avoided when providers engage, educate, and empower their patients and those who care for them through an empathic lens.

Empathy will break down barriers and build better relationships, which will foster better care and result in healthier communities and better outcomes.

THE BUSINESS OF HEALTHCARE

Without empathy in the business of healthcare, our patients are not the only ones getting lost in the system. Oddly enough, as healthcare marketers, providers, and researchers, we're also lost in the system right alongside the patients we've abandoned. We've lost sight of the significance of the patient in our development of effective therapies and meaningful communication strategies. We've failed to see that the answers we seek as marketers often come from the patients and related stakeholders themselves.

Genuine patient conversations have been lost due to over-regulation, protective protocols, lack of curiosity, and inadequate innovation. Sadly, these conversations have been replaced with technology-centered, disconnected checklists and automated tech solutions that are borne from the lowest common denominator in terms of relevance and applicability. We've undermined our ability to develop a truly patient-centered healthcare system because we've eroded our trusted patient relationships with technological solutions that are cold, impersonal, and potentially ineffective. As marketers, we're relationship builders, but we've lost our way. Tech (defined here as a digital interface) is not a silver bullet—but relevancy and human engagement just might be.

We may be on the side of the healthcare industrialists as marketers, but we have a unique opportunity to bridge the gap between the patient and their healthcare with effective communication. Whether we're the owners or strategists within a marketing agency, a director of marketing for a hospital or health system, marketing professionals at a pharmaceutical, or patient education advocates at a life sciences company, we have the tools to change the efficacy of the entire system. And in order to illuminate a better path forward within that system, we have to understand and know how to use the protocols and tools found in ethnography, anthropology, and design thinking.

THE REBIRTH OF HEALTHCARE MARKETING

After years of wrestling with the usefulness and value of tech as an effective way to engage with, educate, and empower patients, the pendulum is swinging in the other direction. We're finally starting to see the full value of the patient voice in crafting our strategies. This rebirth in healthcare marketing is a result of years of evolution in how we connect with, understand, and communicate with the very people we're charged to take care of—marketing is more of a human science than one might imagine. Human understanding is the starting point, and the path we're on goes back a half-century or more. We have experience and a foundation of capabilities that's ready to champion a few fresh tools into the way we work as healthcare marketers.

Ethnography and design thinking are the tools driving this rebirth. Now more than ever before, this combination of science and innovation is the perfect solution to framing effective marketing strategies within the context of a patient-centered healthcare system. Together, these two tools will help us create better messaging of products and services tailored to the needs of patients. This will be achieved through the cultivation and championing of better relationships amongst everyone in the healthcare transaction, from providers and patients to hospitals and pharmaceutical companies.

Ethnography is one of several tools in the design thinking toolbox and is, in my opinion, the most important. As a marketing framework, design thinking offers an interdisciplinary approach to truly understanding the experience of a target audience so that problems are solved with innovative plans and effective communication strategies. It's a methodology for creative problem-solving that prioritizes the interests of everyone involved.

In our estimation, the best design thinkers in healthcare are those who are thinking and acting like cultural anthropologists. These are the researchers and design thinking practitioners who are determined to meet with patients and families on their own turf to truly observe what's happening at ground level and from the insider's perspective. They are also the ones focused on deeply understanding and systematically mapping the patient's functional, cognitive, and emotional experiences along the illness (and care delivery) journey; properly documenting and then contextualizing their research findings; and ultimately aligning their solution design with the most critical needs and values of the patient and stakeholder audience. As you will see in this book, patient experiences, marketing and business outcomes, and—more importantly—healthcare outcomes can significantly improve with the implementation of ethnography and design thinking as the foundation for your marketing and patient engagement strategy.

If we begin our journey by listening to the patient's story, we can formulate tailored engagement, education, and treatment plans that provide patients the tools they need to become both educated *and* empowered in the most important business in which they will ever invest. Ultimately, the messaging and experiences that we enable providers to offer their patients should empower patients toward a higher level of competency and accountability in their own healthcare. This is the promise of design—this is the reason for the rebirth.

PATIENT CENTRICITY

Clearly, patient centricity is not a new concept. One of its first shining moments appeared in the middle of the twentieth century, thanks to Enid Balint, a British psychoanalyst and social welfare worker. She coined the term "patient-centered medicine" before phrases like "patient-centered care" and "shared decision-making" and "value-based" entered the nomenclature of healthcare strategists. Enid and her husband, Michael Balint, were among the first social researchers to connect the biomedical status of a patient with their emotional health.

Balint sought to persuade other doctors to embrace psychoanalysis as a mandatory step in patient treatment. But, while it was a sound argument, it was not embraced by practitioners at the time. In fact, in the late 1970s, the trend was for doctors to only focus on physical diseases they could see. Addiction, depression, cultural nuances, and social anomalies were seen as separate from physical disease, and physicians rarely considered them an integrated healthcare issue.

We've made progress since then. The "burden of disease" and "burden of treatment," as many healthcare practitioners now refer to it, involves physical, mental, and behavioral components of a patient's lived experience. The Affordable Care Act and other recent healthcare reforms place a tremendous premium on patient understanding and satisfaction. The 21st Century Cures Act, passed into law in 2016, approaches pharmaceutical product development with a patient focus, pulling the patient voice into the conversation. Great stuff and significantly important to the notion of how we marketers might approach our trade.

As healthcare marketing, education, and brand professionals, our shining moment and chance to make a difference is now. Without patient centricity as our bedrock, brands fall flat, and educational messaging is ineffective. The patient story is powerful and compelling. When we take the time to listen, it can be life-changing. Listening is not about processing and analyzing the story through an app or database. It's about analyzing it at the human level where open, empathic conversations provide the groundwork for more relevant messaging that engages, educates, empowers, and champions the human condition.

THE FIRST STEPS

One of the hallmark traits amongst us Homo sapiens is that we progress, whether we seek out opportunities for growth, or we subconsciously advance as a species. Growth—and improvement—means adopting new philosophies and challenging old ones. This is what I hope you learn from this book.

As you read, I hope you challenge any old ideas, formulas,

or theories about what healthcare marketing and strategy is. I hope that you look at what it could be when viewed through the lenses of curiosity, design, and, above all, stakeholder empathy. My goal is that you understand the value of a patient-centered approach in clinical education, brand and commercialization strategies, internal stakeholder communications, and healthcare marketing as a whole. There's greater potential for innovative change if we learn to embrace a new way of looking at the stakeholders in healthcare and recognize that they have a lot to share with us.

Finally, my hope is that this book ignites within you the same passion for anthropology that I share with my colleagues and clients. Anthropology and design thinking go hand in hand. With this book, you'll learn about the tools and protocols that design thinkers use in the healthcare space to uncover the most innovative, impactful solutions possible.

CHAPTER 1

H2H HEALTHCARE MARKETING

As marketers, we are used to the terms business-to-business (B2B) and business-to-consumer (B2C)... the time has come for healthcare marketers to champion a more elegant focus, the human-to-human focus.

BRIAN SHAKLEY, PARTNER AT LIFT

It's an understatement to say that healthcare, as an industry, is in the midst of profound evolutionary influences. Every industry evolves, but the healthcare industry is evolving along with the species who are charged with championing it. These days, we find ourselves refocusing after years and years of operating with a physician-centered mindset. Many of the people I work with are starting to realize the wisdom behind the concept that the patient's point of view is where the best solutions in medicine start.

Patient centricity, person centricity, human centricity, stakeholder centricity (call it what you will) is not a new concept. It seems simple enough when we think about it as a human-focused approach to medical science and care delivery, but the variables in that short definition make the idea of centricity a complicated topic.

What does a human focus in medicine really mean? A variety of characteristics make us human, from our ability to invent and develop language to how we connect with one another on an empathic level. It's complicated, and understanding the words, images, behaviors, and symbols of a person's reality are crucial to truly discerning who they are and what they value in terms of health and well-being. At the heart of patient centricity is an understanding of what I would call the "human aspect."

The complexity of the human aspect of healthcare doesn't come in the definition; it comes in the process of understanding. Our understanding of medical science changes with each generation as we focus on what healthcare means to us, what it means to our patients, and what it can be for all of us in the future.

It's true that the fields of medicine, healthcare, and well-being are not a straightforward subject; however, a better understanding of how medicine and patient care have evolved through the years yields a clearer idea of patient centricity and its place in healthcare today and in the future.

A REVOLUTION BEGINS

As discussed in the introduction, when British psychoanalyst Enid Balint introduced the idea of patient-centered medicine in the 1960s, she proposed a different way of looking at illness and the human body. Rather than focusing on the section of the body impacted by disease, she suggested that the medical community consider the whole patient first. She believed that a patient's history, as well as their mental and emotional health, had an impact on their physical state and overall well-being.

Balint persuaded health practitioners to use a whole-person medical approach that incorporates what is essentially psychotherapy. At the time, the practice of medicine was in what we called the "biomedical" phase of its evolution. Most doctors relied on their scientific training to diagnose and treat patients, and the psychological history and status of a patient was rarely considered. In fact, the idea of even paying attention to psychological or sociological components was frowned upon—even shunned. But with Balint's emergence, some doctors were already finding value in the new theory that connected the psychological with the scientific.

In a 1968 gathering of the American Psychiatric Association,

Balint shared her paper, *"The Possibility of Patient-Centered Medicine,"* with those in attendance. In the paper, Balint presents a case study about "Dr. C" and his patient, "Mrs. Grace R.," a woman in her thirties suffering from chronic tension headaches. Mrs. Grace visited Dr. C looking for pain relief with little hope of eliminating the headaches. She believed the headaches were caused by the noisy environment at her work as a machine operator in a power station.

Rather than taking a purely biomedical approach, Dr. C extensively interviewed Mrs. Grace to determine the cause of her headaches. He found that Mr. Grace was Mrs. Grace's second husband and that he was a passive man, much older than her. The two had not been intimate in years; in fact, Mrs. Grace dreaded the entire subject. She chose not to have children because she, herself, had not experienced a stable childhood growing up as a foster child.

I view Mrs. Grace's case as one of the earliest examples of healthcare's use of the kind of in-depth interviewing techniques deployed by modern-day healthcare anthropologists. Dr. C used more than just the scientific tools he had available to him to diagnose Mrs. Grace with anxiety and depression. Instead, he relied on his interviews, in combination with the scientific tools, to determine a framework for her reality and behavior. He determined that her mental state had physical repercussions, and in place of medication, he used Balint's recommended tools of social work and psychotherapy to help Mrs. Grace work through her feelings.

After a few weeks of treatment, little had changed for Mrs. Grace. She still battled frequent headaches, and her depression had a strong hold on her behavior and emotions. Over time, though, and without traditional biomedical intervention, Mrs. Grace was happier and healthier without the help of medication. She had fewer headaches, and she decided to quit her job to spend her time doing things she enjoyed. While she needed to continue her psychological treatment, her patient journey—void of medication, biomedical interventions, and quick remedies—was significant for the medical community. Whether they chose to acknowledge it is a different story.

CRACKS IN THE SYSTEM

As Mrs. Grace worked through her sexual anxiety, Balint's theory of patient-oriented medicine struggled to find its foothold in England. The United States in the late 1970s, for all its revolutions in the decade prior, wasn't much more progressive in the areas of science, medicine, and the incorporation of psychoanalysis—at least as far as the patient was concerned.

No matter the country, there was a disdainful undercurrent of psychosocial perspectives in the science of medicine.

The medical and scientific communities felt that doctors should focus on "real diseases" rather than the psychological rabbit holes of emotional well-being and behavioral health. The general sentiment of the medical community toward the incorporation of behavioral science within their profession was to keep them separate from one another. As doctor, psychiatrist, and psychotherapy advocate George L. Engel put it in his article "The Need for a New Medical Model: A Challenge for Biomedicine," "a disentanglement of the ordinary elements of disease from the psychosocial elements of human malfunction," is what they were championing. The majority of physicians desperately wanted to keep the "ordinary" physical aspects of disease from the challenging psychosocial world of disorders.

Understanding a patient's burden of disease and their lived experience was not a priority for the medical community forty years ago. These character disorders, addictions, depressions, cultural realities, and social anomalies were not seen as treatable mental illnesses or relevant to disease. Instead, they were viewed as psychiatric disorders or cultural curiosities that were not the concern of medical physicians. After all, the dominant medical model of the late twentieth century was the biomedical model, and as beneficial as it was for those in the medical community who embraced science, it failed the patient overall. Instead, it created a crisis of uncertainty that left little room for the social, behavioral, and cultural dimensions of illness. The biomedical model mandated that illness should be treated with a strictly scientific point of view, independent of psychological or social considerations. As doctors and healthcare workers followed the narrow course of biomedicine, the *whole* patient was abandoned.

There were cracks in the medical theory of how healthcare practitioners approached patient care and applied biomedical principles, yet few saw them in the late seventies. Those who did recognize the gaps in the prevailing theory of the day were the social scientists. At the other end of the debate were the naysayers, comprised of clinical scientists. Many saw the social scientists as heretics who questioned the biomedical model's ultimate truth. Rather than buying into this popular model, social scientists believed that diseases related to human behavior *could* be brought into the clinical realm and treated with clinical principles. Thus began a crisis of uncertainty in healthcare—and opened the door to what is now known as ethnomedical science.

ETHNOMEDICAL SCIENCE AND THE BIOPSYCHOSOCIAL MODEL

Ethnomedical science stands on the premise that behavioral science is not only related to biological science, but both are inextricably intertwined. Those who agree with this stance deny that the psychosocial element interferes with patient care. They also recognize that the psychological characteristics of a patient influence their biomedical functions. From their beginning in the latter part of the twentieth century, ethnomedical scientists advocated for this new way of thinking in the medical community. Ultimately, they brought medicine to life—or rather—they brought life to medicine.

With this new understanding, behavioral therapy was closer to universal acceptance as a window into a patient's well-being. Physicians and psychotherapists became one, assuming the role of "patient educator." Clinical research, primary care, and the psychosocial elements of the patient converged into a new model of medicine called the biopsychosocial model. Suddenly, the patient—the whole human—was squarely in the middle of the healthcare transaction where he or she should have been from the very beginning.

Patients finally had a voice, and each patient's opinion had a foothold in the healthcare space. You might even say that the biopsychosocial model in medicine provided a bedrock for patient centricity. Whether it's called patient-centered care, person-centered care, or a stakeholder-centered model, it's human centricity. It's Balint's patient-oriented healthcare. It's understanding how social factors combine with physiological and psychological functions to create a whole person with symptoms and treatment needs. More than anything, it's understanding that patients are people—and if we're not operating with this notion in mind as we develop educational materials, treatment options, and even new medications—we're starting in the wrong place.

HEALTHCARE: UNDERDESIGNED AND OVERREGULATED

We're on the brink of major change in healthcare and healthcare marketing, and it isn't too soon. We have regulations for every aspect, from care protocols to stakeholder engagement requirements. Impactful solutions, designed thoughtfully and effectively, are scarce. The disarray we're working with will continue to evolve for years to come. But we're headed in the right direction with human-centered health initiatives that enable us to design more effective patient-engagement programs and experiences.

As seen from the last forty years in healthcare, paradigm shifts don't happen overnight. In my work as a healthcare anthropologist and strategist at LIFT, which is our healthcare insights and marketing strategy agency, I talk to a variety of healthcare, science, research, and marketing professionals daily. Fortunately, I've seen a promising evolution of strategic thinking over the past few years. I've also encountered many a fresh face interested in digging deeper and looking at strategy through the eyes of the patient. Let me share a few case studies:

HEALTH NETWORKS

A colleague, Paul Szablowski, was the senior vice president of communications and image at a large health system. He was responsible for leading public relations, physician and employee communications, and branding and advertising for the health system. When I met Paul, he was seeking a more innovative marketing strategy across the Texas Health Resources (THR) enterprise. He viewed healthcare as the most overregulated and underdesigned industry in the world, and he believed in a better way to leverage his marketing and communications investments.

THR serves a large population of uninsured and under-served patients. Paul was interested in learning how the hospitals in his system were relevant to these communities and wanted to engage them before they reached his doorstep. He believed that investing in population health management initiatives and community engagement programs—educating and empowering healthy behavior—would make better use of his marketing investments and thereby cultivate healthier communities across the THR footprint.

To that end, Paul wanted to create a culture of human understanding among his marketing strategists. He viewed design thinking as the perfect lens through which to accomplish such a vision. To make his vision a reality, Paul asked one of our senior designers and me to envision an interactive program that would cultivate a culture of empathy within the organization's marketing and brand groups.

The resulting program was the perfect mix of healthcare and marketing knowledge combined with extreme stakeholder empathy and the tools of design thinking. The program we designed for Paul aimed to create an environment where marketing and clinical professionals could interact with various stakeholders in a safe environment and explore service line and community needs through the eyes of the stakeholders. Including the patient at the center of the healthcare transaction set a new bar for how business and marketing strategies would be crafted.

THE PHARMACEUTICAL INDUSTRY

Pharmaceutical companies are connecting with patients at ground level. Take, for example, the 21st Century Cures Act, which was enacted by Congress in December 2016. Through this legislation, novel medical products and products with new indications can receive FDA review, potential approval, and ultimately go to market faster—in some cases, six months faster—if the regulatory package contains evidence detailing the patient experience using the product or therapy. This ensures that the patients' voices become a part of the drug approval decisions, complementing perfectly the data from clinical trials. It also puts the patient squarely at the center of asset and brand development.

For patients, this means better individual and clinical outcomes and improved patient experiences. For healthcare companies, it can lead to better alignment with patient realities. It's interesting to note that, while healthcare providers have been focusing on patient-centered initiatives and innovations for many years, pharmaceutical companies are now beginning to see the benefits that can be gained from the rich source of knowledge that is the patient's voice. Hearing and understanding the patient voice allows companies to develop more effective products.

At LIFT, we were contacted by a global pharmaceutical company preparing for Phase 3 study and subsequent regulatory filings. Their desire was to leverage the voice of psoriasis patients as a component of their trials and regulatory package. LIFT was asked to design an ethnographic study to interview psoriasis patients and clinical trial participants to gain a better understanding of the patient's quality of life, burden of disease, lived experience, and other aspects of the disease and treatment. We were specifically tasked to assess each patient's satisfaction, concerns, fatigue, sexual health, family issues, and their burdens of suffering from psoriasis.

LIFT designed a multifaceted study incorporating a series of tools intended to highlight the lived experience. We wanted to document the voice of the patient for potential use in the ensuing regulatory package and to support brand development. The study design included ethnography as well as elicitation and a few design thinking tools like journey mapping, expectation mapping, scenario presentation, and role playing. Through our efforts, we sought to effectively understand the concerns and needs of the participants in the study.

Instead of relying solely on highly selective, less generalizable, traditional clinical trials, the FDA has begun to show an interest in understanding the patient experience when it comes to the actual clinical use of drugs, biologics, devices, and other medical products. With this increased interest, there is now a greater focus on the patient experience as a way to gain better clarity around diseases and the lived experience. Consequently, healthcare companies are engaging with patients early in the development process to ensure an in-depth understanding of the burden of disease, unmet needs, and the complete treatment experience from the patient's point of view.

MEDICAL DEVICES

Velano Vascular is an amazing upstart device company. I met its CEO, Eric Stone, when his company was in the early stages of marketing PIVO, a device for drawing blood without the use of a needle. Through the use of a peripherally inserted catheter (PIC) with both a long and short tube, blood is collected pain-free and without procedural issues that have historically plagued the use of PICs in blood draws. While they're the most common medical procedure in the world, blood draws can be a challenging undertaking for the phlebotomist and a traumatic event for the patient, especially for children and seniors. With the use of PIVO, hospital patients can sleep through the night while nurses collect multiple blood samples, allowing more efficiency in healthcare and less stress for everyone involved.

Eric came to LIFT because he wanted to understand the patient experience and how to communicate the story of his product and brand to potential customers and investors. Ethnography interested him, so we applied this approach and implemented a study. We headed out into the environment where the device was piloted to better understand the people whose lives were affected by it. We spoke with advocacy organizations, patients and their caregivers, nurses and doctors, and CEOs and chief medical officers to learn everything we could about their reality. It wasn't long before we were able to conclude that Velano Vascular offered a highly desirable product for the patient, the phlebotomist, *and* the healthcare system—a product that incorporated a patient-centered philosophy at the pivotal point of care.

Subsequently, LIFT was able to tell the Velano and PIVO story in a compelling manner—leveraging the voices of myriad stakeholders to demystify their offering while highlighting the value to the various stakeholders most notably impacted. The resulting brand story and supporting marketing and education programs have helped Velano gain significant traction in their commercialization journey. LIFT continues to support Velano as they expand market share by continuing to tell their story through the eyes (and in the words) of the patient and healthcare providers most impacted by their novel technology.

HOSPITAL AND HEALTHCARE SYSTEM

One of our first forays into patient-centered marketing for hospitals and health networks was with a small independent hospital system in Delaware called Beebe Healthcare. At the time, Beebe was refreshing the voice of their women's healthcare service line. Alex Sydnor, the vice president of strategy and marketing at Beebe, was interested in a new approach to this initiative—seeking to determine how his system connected with and activated women consumers in his markets.

The biggest challenge for Beebe was a lack of understanding around the local cultural drivers of health behavior in women. Alex viewed ethnography and design thinking as fresh and powerful tools, which he and his staff could use to reimagine how his system would frame their marketing strategy for a service line targeted at a diverse swath of patients.

At Alex's request, LIFT set up a design studio on the Beebe campus. We deployed an anthropologist and an ethnographic filmmaker into the community to conduct empirical research and document the lives of the women of Beebe. While the ethnographers were in the field capturing a high-fidelity picture of the women in the community, a LIFT design team was interacting with staff, patients, and community stakeholders in a design studio. The idea was to apply the tools and protocols of design thinking to understand current state realities and begin the process of envisioning a more stakeholder-centric future state. LIFT was able to leverage ethnography as a cornerstone component in understanding the community and patient journey. We then utilized design thinking methodologies to craft messaging that elevated the voice of Beebe to align with the values and beliefs of the various communities served in women's health.

All this activity produced a trove of valuable data and content. We were able to use this data in framing a creative strategy that was grounded in the voices and realities of the women and clinical and community stakeholders that Beebe was seeking to connect with and empower. The resulting marketing strategies have created a continuous experience that extends beyond the four walls of the hospital. Beebe has successfully moved beyond sick care and into the realm of well-being through education. They've articulated a voice for women's health services that resonates with a broad range of patient personas and cohorts. Together, they're unified in realizing Beebe's desire to become a health improvement organization as well as a place for folks to come when they're sick.

Beebe has identified the unique manner in which to speak to the women in *its* community. It has successfully developed a strategy for both online and offline tactics that inspires and moves women to take a more active role in their health and well-being. Above all, it has created a continuous experience between itself and the women it serves. The voice Beebe has developed for women's health services speaks to women as a whole—but also to each of the user groups.

LIFT has leveraged the voice and face of the Beebe community, which is embodied by real patients, to design messaging and content for virtually every channel imaginable—from a custom consumer magazine to a multifaceted digital hub supported by a robust multichannel marketing program. Our use of ethnography and design thinking has facilitated several excellent and successful campaigns and programs that continue today to support the Beebe vision.

These are a few examples of the power of a little ethnography and some design thinking to develop a deep understanding of who the brand community is and how best to engage with them. The tools of design continue to help these clients and set the stage for engagement and marketing strategies grounded in a language that's relevant to each unique strategic application. These examples illustrate that understanding the consumer and how they intersect with the brand provides an evidence-based approach to how we shape our voice. They also identify to what extent we believe we can impact the consumer experience for better outcomes on both sides of the transaction. A win-win that would not be possible without design or anthropology.

WHERE DO WE GO FROM HERE?

After nearly fifty years exploring the meaning and role of patient centricity across virtually every domain of healthcare, it's clear that we're making great progress. Healthcare is a human endeavor. As marketers, we have an obligation to leverage human understanding into the work we do in engaging, educating, and empowering patients (and other stakeholders). The biopsychosocial model provides compelling guardrails for how we can approach every aspect of interacting with the people who make up every healthcare transaction.

A patient's understanding of their own health—and the decisions they make regarding their health—matters more than ever before. By changing our focus from a biomedical approach to a biopsychosocial view, we have a more human-centered framework for innovation and change. As marketers, we know we have to engage with and educate our customers. In doing so, we empower behaviors intended to nurture a more competent patient and care-giver. Cultural and social considerations are important in understanding a patient's story. And when we understand each patient's story, patient care improves for everyone.

CHAPTER 2

GETTING IT RIGHT, SO WE DON'T GET IT WRONG

It is clear that culture does matter in the clinic. Cultural factors are critical to diagnosis, treatment, and care. They shape health-related beliefs, behaviors, and values.

ARTHUR KLEINMAN, AUTHOR OF
THE ILLNESS NARRATIVES

Marketing and communication professionals play an important role in building and maintaining a patient-centered brand. Understanding patients begins outside the walls of the healthcare setting. What we learn from these patients provides a strong foundation for impactful messaging that results in improved clinical *and* business outcomes. I believe that engaging and relevant interactions will educate and empower consumer competency, which will create a higher level of personal accountability. This connection will lead to each patient playing a more active role in his or her health and well-being.

As healthcare marketers, we're in an unambiguous position to impact the health of the consumer while successfully delivering on strategy and financial demands. Our first priority should be understanding, engaging with, educating, and empowering patients. By approaching our professions through the lens of human understanding, we can then collaborate with the multiple stakeholders to develop a nuanced understanding of our brands, which competitors will find enviable.

Championing a patient-focused marketing and communication strategy is a significant commitment. As with any commitment, there are both challenges and benefits that come from leading the way with this type of strategy and plan. Despite the challenges, our objective is clear—to empower better health through messaging and engagement. Understanding each individual stakeholder as intimately as possible is an important first step in reaching that objective. Knowing where to focus and knowing the hurdles we face in terms of behavior change is equally important.

As marketers, we're keen to move behavior and to cultivate

trust that results in a positive outcome for our brands and, more importantly, for the patients we seek to care for. In my work as a healthcare marketing strategist and anthropologist, I've found four considerations that are foundational to any patient-centered marketing strategy—linguistics, literacy, competency, and accountability. Engaging with patients is a journey of its own, and these four touchstones are, in a small way, sequential. Not understanding them will put the marketer at a disadvantage.

LINGUISTICS

Disseminating health information has been a cornerstone of marketing and patient education for many years—and that is likely not going to change anytime soon. Print, digital, video, and experiential content is the foundation of patient engagement and education—all intended to empower behavior. I think about of the role of language in healthcare as a function of linguistic anthropology, which is the interdisciplinary study and understanding of how language influences social life. In the case of healthcare, it's how language can influence patient and stakeholder behavior.

Language makes cultures come to life. It shapes interactions and behavior, and it plays an important role in our social identity and ideology. Our language shapes our reality. Despite our personal story, our background, and our culture, each of us intersects with others within, what we call at LIFT, the intersections of common human truths. It's our responsibility, as marketers, to understand these truths and to use appropriate linguistic narrative as a vital tool to focus our messaging.

As communication professionals, we need to be sensitive to the linguistic and cultural aspects of how we engage, educate, and empower the communities we want to influence. Hospitals and health networks have struggled with these aspects of patient relations for years. As marketers, however, we have a unique opportunity to understand the patient reality and to offer value in messaging that is as beneficial to the patient as it is to the brand.

Think about it. What we do is important—we use language to influence behavior. It goes beyond a catchy design or an appealing phrase. Our words must be readable, relatable, and approachable, drawing in patients and empowering them to play an active role in their own health and well-being. Print, digital, and experiential content inform our engagement strategies and assists in patient education.

Clients hire us to craft the voice of their brands and therapies, and to show patients how a treatment can impact them. Translation is important, but cultural appropriateness is one of the most challenging and powerful areas of linguistics.

To illustrate the importance of the words we use, let's look at psoriasis—a lifelong autoimmune disease that leaves patients with scaly, torturous rashes. Sufferers live with chronic pain that is both physically *and* mentally exhausting, meeting each new day with swollen, achy legs and rashes sometimes covering even the bottoms of their feet.

Biologic therapies are typically the only relief for these patients. If our mission is to develop communication protocols for psoriasis support in southern California, we must understand the point of view of both the doctor and the patient in southern California. Marketing must account for social and cultural diversity and be sensitive to both the physician's medical philosophy as well as the background of their patients. Southern California is known to serve multiple cultural communities and, therefore, all communication should, as much as possible, be tailored to the primary language of the audience, including the colloquialisms and cultural nuances that shape it.

Educating patients requires more expertise than simply knowing about the disease. To engage our patients and empower them, we must understand how their language intersects with their cultural beliefs. Connecting with the patient enables us to earn their trust and build a more secure relationship with them, leading to a better marketing outcome and more successful solutions.

LITERACY

Literacy relates to the patient's ability to read and comprehend messages and information. Even when our message is tailored to our audience and presented in a linguistically thoughtful way, we still face communication challenges. Every day, patients are handed forms to complete and brochures to read. According to the Journal of Medical Internet Research article, "Health Literacy and Health Information Technology Adoption: The Potential for a New Digital Divide," patients with low health literacy are less likely to use health information technology like apps and portals. If they actually do use them, they rarely find them easy to use or beneficial. Oftentimes, patients are almost required to be highly literate in order to engage with our healthcare system and receive the full benefit.

We can define literacy in healthcare as a patient's ability to read, write, speak, compute, and solve problems related to their healthcare. It's how they comprehend and act on the information provided to them. Healthcare is already difficult to navigate for patients—imagine lacking the basic tools necessary to take the first step in this challenge.

According to the United States Department of Health and Human Services, the majority of Americans are at an intermediate level of health literacy, and seventy-seven million adults have basic or below basic health literacy.

This means that millions of Americans struggle with the most fundamental aspects of healthcare—from completing applications and reading health advisories before medical tests, to communicating issues to physicians and understanding instructions for self-care after a procedure. We're not talking about just patients, either. Health illiteracy is an issue for all stakeholders in the healthcare transaction, including clinical staff and caregivers.

Literate patients are healthier patients. Those with low literacy levels are less compliant with their treatment, and many even fail to tell their healthcare practitioners of their struggles in the first place. When they do follow a prescription or treatment protocol, they make more errors, resulting in a greater chance that they'll suffer the consequences. In cases of chronic diseases like hypertension, asthma, HIV, or diabetes, low-literacy patients know significantly less about their condition than a high-literacy patient, and likely know very little about how to manage it.

Health literacy is more than just lacking the ability to read. Patients who struggle to comprehend written information have a difficult time following instructions, and they may even struggle with math skills. Healthcare involves calculating cholesterol and blood sugar levels, measuring medications, and analyzing nutrition labels—all feats that are difficult for patients who possess a lower level of literacy skills.

There is often a tremendous gap between what we communicate to the healthcare consumer and what they understand. How valuable is our communication and how effective is our treatment if our message isn't received? These are patients and caregivers who rely on the system to nurture well-being and provide guidance for themselves and the loved ones they care for. Well-being is a joint venture between the patient, the community in which they reside, and the system that supports them. As healthcare marketers, we're part of that community and system they depend on. It's our job to communicate in a way that provides the most positive outcome possible.

By addressing these two areas of linguistics and literacy first, we lay the foundation for a more successful patient and caregiver experience. It allows us to create and deliver messaging that's aligned to the needs of the patient. And by engaging with customers in a language that is relevant to them, and on the appropriate literacy level, we set the stage for a positive encounter. Relevancy in marketing is more than subject matter focus—it's about connecting with consumers in a voice that the patient finds engaging, understandable, and of interest. If we accomplish this, we'll have a captive audience who will be more open to learning and more empowered—and an empowered patent is more likely to become a competent patient.

Delivering brand messages at the appropriate literacy level is paramount. In doing so, we're nurturing competency in how the patient receives and processes messages. But there's more to competency than linguistics. The competence I'm referring to is a more whole spectrum of consumer competency—not just one that relates to how a consumer interacts with and uses our healthcare system and brands to their optimal advantage.

Elevating consumer competency is very important in the evolution of our healthcare system. As marketers, we have an opportunity to empower consumers to play an active role in their health and well-being. As I've stated previously, an important role we play as marketers is the role of educating. An educated patient is more empowered, and an empowered patient is more likely to be a competent patient.

Competence in healthcare is another area of focus that, when empowered, adds to the foundation of a patient-centered brand. In the process of cultivating consumer competency, we must understand the culture and beliefs of the individual or group we seek to empower. In order to impact positively, we have to be culturally relevant. This bedrock of relevancy can be a powerful base for better outcomes. Consumer and cultural competence is an active process—one that requires the development of skills necessary to effectively engage in cross-cultural situations.

When a patient or caregiver struggles with making reasonable decisions about the appropriate path to improved health, we assess their health competence, or their ability to manage treatment. We can break down competence into cognitive, media, and instrumental competence.

Cognitive competence is a patient's capacity to understand information presented to them. Media competence is their ability to not only understand messaging, but to analyze it and provide feedback. The media-competent consumer understands their treatment options, considers their support system with their medical staff and family, and they combine this information with the guidance and educational materials provided by the healthcare provider—whether that's a hospital, pharmaceutical company, or product manufacturer.

Instrumental competence is one step further in critical thinking. It requires a patient to make good decisions based on what they learn. This is a tangible type of competence where the patient, as a decision-maker, helps create their own treatment and healthcare experience. They take what they learn, make an informed decision, and commit to their treatment plan.

The competent patient combines cognitive, media, and instrumental competence to take charge of their health. They become a responsible and accountable patient who's able to choose the best treatment for themselves. They engage in productive health behaviors because they understand their condition and the resources available to them.

Competency leads to a higher level of personal account-ability, which is another crucial domain of human behavior that can add tremendous value to the system.

ACCOUNTABILITY

Accountability is such a powerful thing. Self-motivated, competent consumers are generally aware of their surroundings and will ordinarily take some personal responsibility for their actions and their own well-being. By understanding the patient's point of view and engaging with them in language that is relatable and relevant, we're nurturing a higher level of awareness and understanding about their own situation. That higher level of understand-ing leads to an empowered consumer.

Our entire healthcare system, from a financial and quality of care standpoint, improves when patients are account-able to their own health and well-being. If you increase competency, you have a greater chance of increasing accountability. In healthcare, competent consumers are more likely to play an active role in their own health and well-being and thereby accept some level of accountability in their own clinical outcome. Competent and accountable patients make for better economic outcomes.

If the other barriers in effective communication and patient empowerment are not overcome, patient accountability is nearly impossible to achieve. Patients fail to follow therapy guidelines and are unable to be accountable when the language in marketing and educational material is intellectually inaccessible to them. Sadly, when literacy is a challenge, there's almost no hope that the patient will become competent or responsible. Other factors, such as medication side effects, psychiatric illness, and treatment costs also stand in the way of a patient's overall ability to be responsible for their healthcare.

A brand and marketing strategy that's grounded in an understanding of the patient and focused on the importance of language and literacy inevitably provides a foundation for competence. It's only logical that our messages must nurture competence before we can hold a patient responsible. Responsible patients are those who understand the healthier choices, listen to their physicians, use their therapy as intended, and are compliant with prescriptions and related treatments or therapeutic paths. They want to have a say in their treatment because they understand it. Most importantly, they reward themselves with better treatment outcomes, and they reward the process by costing the system less money. Responsible patients are gladly willing to be held accountable.

A NEW KIND OF STRATEGY

If you consider these four touchstones of strategy—linguistics, literacy, competence, and accountability—as a journey, you can see how getting one right can help get the others right, too. Each area of focus is like a stepping-stone in every patient's healthcare journey. If we, as marketers, understand the consumer and get our language right, and the patient can successfully read what we've written, it will lead to greater consumer competence and patient accountability. Ultimately, it will lead to success for everyone involved in the process. Each one builds on the other, and each one is a valuable, patient-centered strategy.

If we want to connect with those we serve and help them to more fully play an active role in their own healthcare journey, every successful, patient-centered strategy must start with patient understanding. With the help of ethnography, we're able to understand our patients in such a way that all four of these touchstones can be addressed. When we fail to apply ethnography to our brands or marketing strategy, we fail to understand and connect to the very people we're trying to help. Ethnography is not only the key to patient-centered healthcare, it's the process by which we'll help patients become greater advocates of themselves.

CHAPTER 3

ANTHROPOLOGY: EMPATHY AT WORK

*What people say, what people do, and what they say they do
are entirely different things.*

MARGARET MEAD, AMERICAN ANTHROPOLOGIST

In 2006, a group of medical researchers who were interested in public health noticed that Haitian women in a coastal community in Florida had consistently high rates of ovarian cancer. In fact, thirty-eight women out of every 100,000 suffered from the disease. Interviews with the clinical world failed to shed light on the reason, so researchers dug deeper. They used ethnography to focus on the women, immersing themselves in their culture to understand why cervical cancer was so prevalent there.

Their work paid off. Researchers found that the Haitian women's cultural beliefs often prohibited screenings from anyone outside their family or community. Because of this, very few women in the community were tested. With the help of design thinking, the research team created a new process that was culturally sensitive to Haitian beliefs. This process eliminated the need for a pelvic exam in a formal clinic that included physician involvement—details of routine gynecological care that conflicted with their Haitian values of modesty. Using a self-sampler swab in the privacy of their homes, the women were able to receive necessary and effective healthcare in a comfortable setting, honoring their cultural values and protecting them as individuals.

This was an astounding breakthrough, made possible through anthropology and design. The solution placed the power of screening in the hands of the patient while still maintaining test accuracy. The health of an entire community improved, and the new process demonstrated a better allocation of healthcare resources. This is a powerful example of the potential of anthropology in healthcare.

ETHNOGRAPHY: BRIDGING THE GAPS

Ethnography, born from anthropology, is a way of seeing the world through engaging, in-depth field research that produces a holistic view of people and the world around them. Until recently, we've lacked a standard interpretation of how ethnography and anthropology fit into healthcare. Now, understanding a patient's reality and how we can leverage that understanding to build a better system of care and provide better education with marketing is fast becoming as important as technology and science in healthcare.

Many brands claim that they know their customers, but how many truly understand them? The gaps between knowing and understanding prevent us from achieving patient centricity in marketing. Ethnography provides us a framework for empathically engaging with patients and actually listening to them. As a direct result, we're able to use design thinking in a way that bridges these gaps and leads us from simply knowing, to deeply understanding.

Ethnography can be identified as far back as the 1700s, beginning with a man by the name of G.F. Müller, who is known as the father of ethnography. Müller was part of the Russian Kamchatka expeditions where artists, scientists, and historians were tasked with recording the life and nature of the people of the Siberian regions. Ethnography has been further clarified by James Spradley, an influential scholar and prolific writer in the field of ethnography (his books were some of the texts I studied in college). Spradley defined ethnography as the process of learning *about* subjects by learning *from* them. It examines the ways that communities are organized and influenced by the world around them, allowing us to view human behavior from multidimensional perspectives.

With the Kamchatka expeditions, ethnography has its earliest roots in social anthropology, a subset of anthropology that focuses on small communities that share culturally specific beliefs and practices. In healthcare, we can use ethnography for any small-scale research completed in everyday settings. Study groups normally include an average of fifteen participants, although as few as seven yield thematic similarities and conclusive data. Several research methods are used in ethnography, from observation and documentation to cultural probes and elicitation techniques.

One of the most interesting things about ethnography is how the process evolves throughout a single study. It emphasizes the importance of understanding the context of a behavior or belief system so that the subject is understood as a whole person, on both a micro and macro level. With a micro examination, we see a patient's everyday experiences. This enables important insights, but looking at the subject from a broader standpoint allows us to understand cultural formations and societal belief systems that emerge from their interactions.

Ethnography is a powerful tool that yields tremendous insight. It also provides a treasure trove of content and creative bedrock that leads to far superior branding and marketing solution design. It will yield a deeper understanding of the patient and the provider, allowing for greater success in healthcare for everyone involved in the process.

Although the benefits of ethnography may be far more than we can now understand, there are six characteristics that best illuminate the value and power of applied ethnography in healthcare research settings:

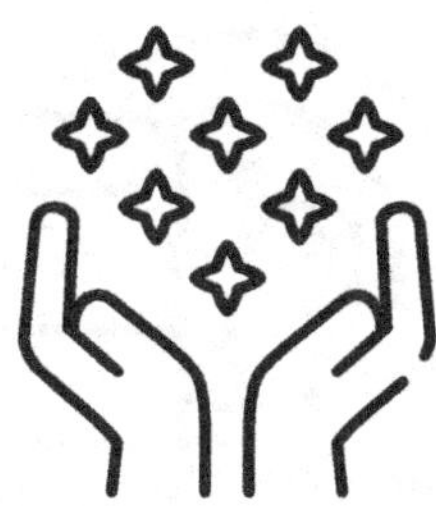

Meaningful—The patient voice is full of substance and meaning. Ethnography helps draw out that voice and provides context around the realities of the patient experience at ground level. This context fuels a deeper understanding and better strategy and design.

Inductive—As we observe, interview, and gain a better understanding of the patient's reality, we can use what we're seeing and learning to allow our thinking to evolve in real time. Ethnography allows new guiding points to emerge in real time, which empowers the researcher to explore more deeply when seeking evidence to support potential conclusions.

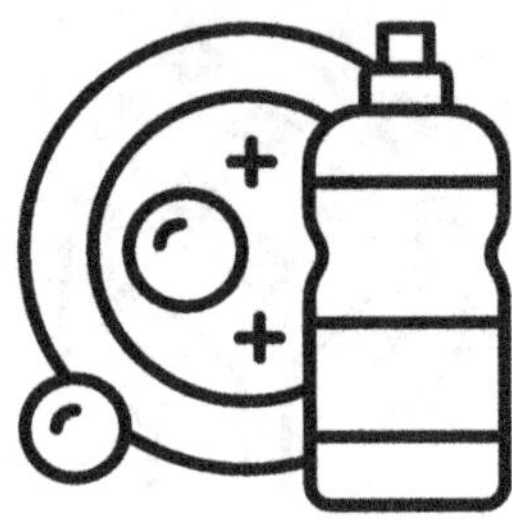

Contextual—Ethnographic studies are always conducted in the context of everyday life where the action occurs. This way, we observe more deeply the meaning or context of a certain reality and how that shapes consumer beliefs and behavior.

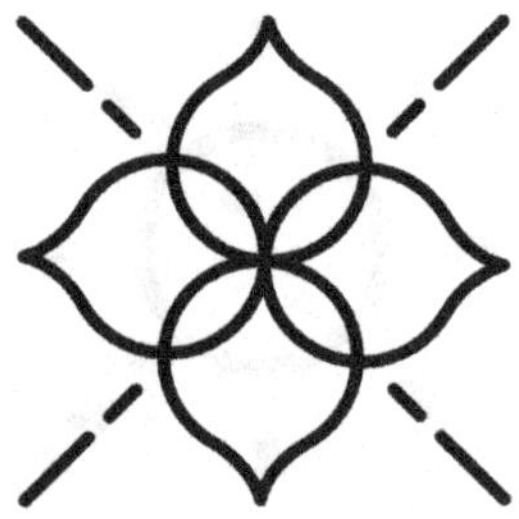

Holistic—The aim of ethnography is always to achieve a comprehensive understanding of human and cultural phenomenon under investigation. Seeking deep insights across the functional, psychological, and emotional levels of reality provides context otherwise unavailable to marketers.

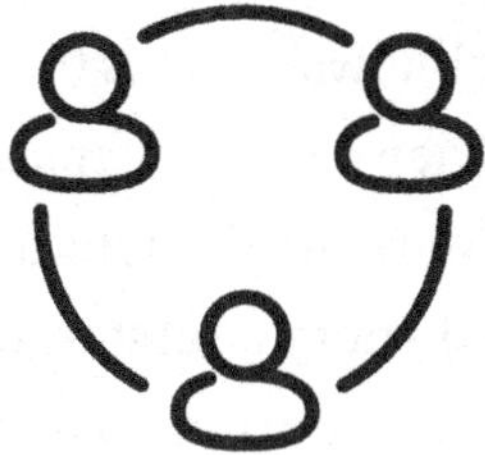

Collaborative—Working collaboratively with patients and their families, caregivers, clinical teams, strategists, design groups, and marketers, ethnography illuminates the human truths necessary to create truly patient-centric brands.

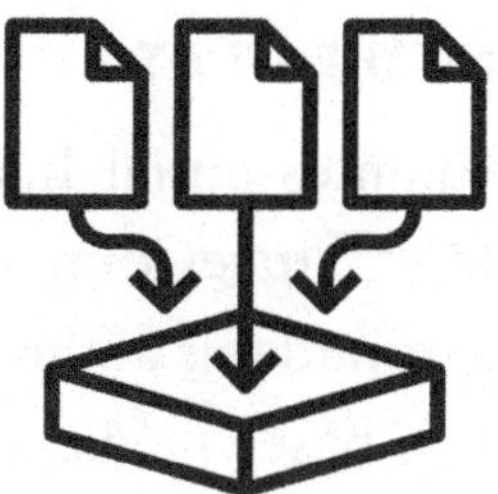

Rigorous—Grounded theory approach requires that we immerse ourselves in the daily lives and routines of the patient. This open-ended research method of studying the world surrounding our patients builds a systematic approach into both data collection and analysis.

I particularly like the quote attributed to Bronisław Malinowski, a Polish anthropologist who taught at Yale. His scholarly writings on the topics of social theory, ethnography, and grounded theory fieldwork have left an indelible—and even controversial—mark on the discipline of anthropology. Malinowski states that "The aim is to penetrate into the worldview of another part of society, or a part of our own, which we really do not know about—or know about, but we really do not understand." This emphasis on understanding is very important. Through the lens of ethnography, we can move from a place of knowing the patient and stakeholders involved in a healthcare transaction to a place of understanding. It's in this place of understanding that we can create effective, patient-focused, impactful, and profitable brands.

THE HUMANS BEHIND THE STUDY

Ethnography is the quintessential, human-to-human science. Rigid scientists and strategic marketing professionals alike are gravitating toward this anthropologic model that some are calling ethno-based medicine.

In healthcare, ethnography positions the patient as the expert. For many patients who participate in an ethnographic study, this is the first time someone from the medical community has asked them to share their daily experiences. Doctors are good at poking and prodding, diagnosing and prescribing, but they rarely listen to a patient describe what it *feels* like to have a disease.

As marketers and healthcare professionals, we're good at talking *at* patients on behalf of a brand, but we sometimes overlook the importance of talking *with* them. We understand the symptoms from the biomedical angle of the patient, but when we skip ethnography, we fail to understand the patient from a biopsychosocial perspective. Patients and adjacent stakeholders are the perfect subjects to interview because they live in the trenches—their illness is an everyday part of their life. Patients provide pure, untainted, expert testimony leading to powerful insight that can otherwise go unnoticed.

Insight is not merely an observation or a piece of data pulled from a patient interaction. An insight is the analysis and interpretation of data that induces meaning and furthers our understanding of a situation, experience, or issue. It's a meaningful connection, an undiscovered truth that surfaces to reveal an unmet need, and a change in perception that causes an intuitive understanding of the reason for a behavior or attitude. Simply stated, an insight is the why behind the what.

IT'S GOOD TO TRY SOMETHING NEW

We're beginning to recognize the value of ethnography as

our healthcare system evolves to champion the patient's and caregiver's point of view. We now *want* to understand more about the experience of the stakeholders—patients, clinicians, and caregivers alike. We want to understand their journey and contextualize their expectations, needs, and motivations. Ethnography is capable of showing us how care decisions and treatment results are influenced by a patient's cultural practices. It also has the potential to reveal ethnocentric assumptions made by physicians and how these assumptions can potentially negatively impact quality of care. Above all, ethnography provides an understanding of the familial aspects of care that are often the most important to the patient.

The impact of ethnography reaches far and wide in the medical community, but we, as healthcare marketers, along with the patients we engage and the brands we champion, are the greatest beneficiaries. With ethnographic research, we know who—and what—we're dealing with. We see our target audience clearly, and we understand the myriad of motivations that drive patients to particular behaviors. This information is invaluable as we create marketing strategies to educate and empower patients, or as we navigate the commercialization landscape in bringing a new product or therapy to market.

We have the privilege to witness real-time experiences in the patient's environment, providing an eye-witness perspective that allows us to resolve issues that previously had no solution. When a psoriasis patient visits a doctor, how often do they discuss the social or psychological impact of their disease? They may talk about the pain and discomfort their rashes cause, but do they mention the toll on their social life because they're too embarrassed to date? Many patients with chronic illnesses like psoriasis struggle with depression and resiliency issues because of the hidden shame and debilitation caused by the disease. With ethnography, we're able to contextualize how we discuss therapy options to find the best course of treatment for the whole patient, rather than just one element of their condition. We learn how to sell empowerment and *real* health, rather than simply a service, product, or drug.

MAPPING: POWERFUL TOOLS FOR BETTER STRATEGIC OUTCOMES

Ethnography offers us a set of supplemental tools that are not traditionally used in qualitative practices like focus groups or patient panels. While ethnography always involves interviews and contextual observation, the exact techniques and instruments we rely on vary depending on the topic and the needs of our clients.

At LIFT, our toolkit includes processes that uncover the context capable of bridging the gap between knowing and understanding. Cultural artifact analysis, mapping, projective techniques, cultural probes, and shadowing are foundational in our mission of uncovering the why behind the what. This search for meaning requires us to dive deeper than we do with traditional qualitative research methods.

One of our most important tools is mapping. As ethnographers and design thinkers, we use mapping to better understand the data we collect and to help illuminate the path forward. Maps provide an excellent visual representation of our findings and realities at ground level. We map contexts, or the various environments in which relevant behavior occurs, along with processes and practices under investigation. We map patient expectations to better understand the important intersections between ourselves and the patient. We also map the patient journey, one of our most popular forms of mapping.

There are several different forms of maps, which are equally important, yet varied in their functions.

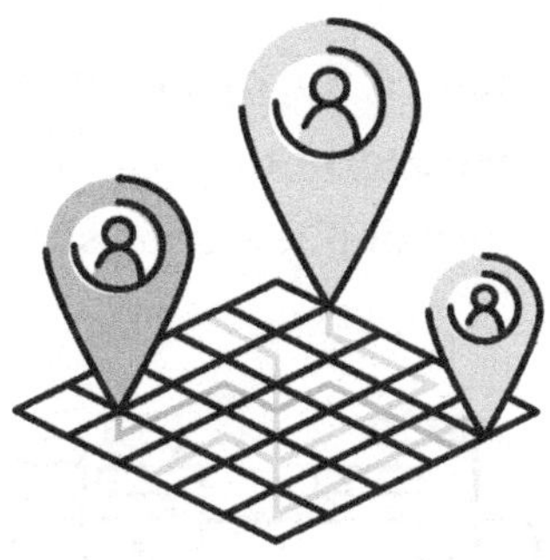

Journey Map

A patient (or stakeholder) journey map is a visual representation of the process that he or she goes through to achieve a goal with your hospital or health system. With the help of a journey map, you can chart stakeholder behavior over time and glean deeper insight into the motivations that drive those behaviors. This will allow you to design and target interventions, experiences, or messages that will influence a positive outcome.

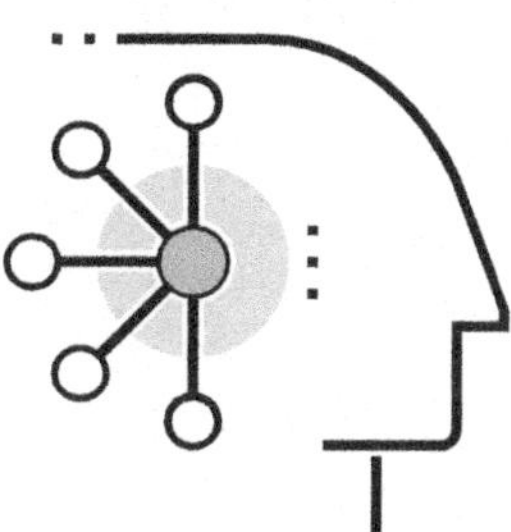

Expectation Map

Expectation mapping is a way of visualizing the patient or stakeholder's emotions within the context of a healthcare or wellness journey. These maps are an excellent way to explore and understand the dynamic and ever-evolving expectations embedded in the vision of what a quality healthcare experience or interaction should feel like.

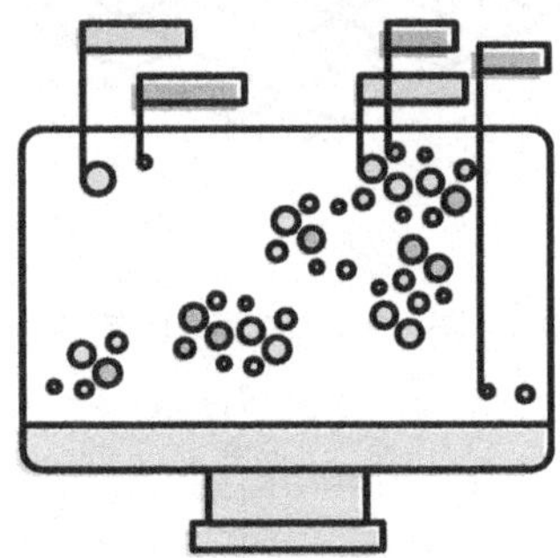

Language Map

A language Map (or more properly called *linguistic map*) is a thematic map illuminating the geographic (or even more locally, internal) distribution of the various speakers of certain languages within your healthcare delivery environment or the community you serve.

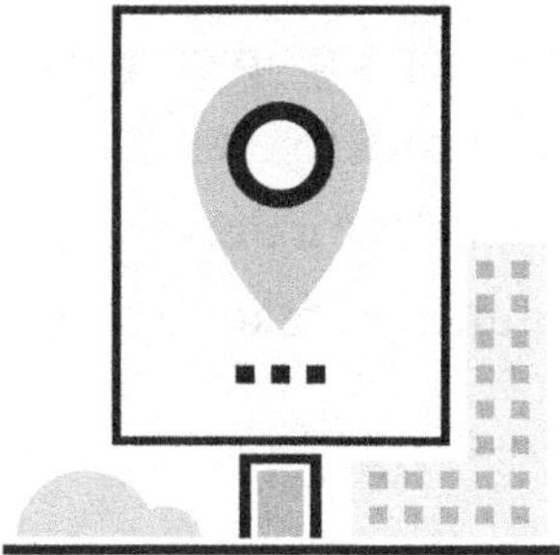

Context Map

A Context Map is the high-level view of a service environment or healthcare ecosystem as a whole. Consisting of various micro—or bounded contexts (at home vs. in a clinic), the collection of bounded contexts fits within a formal healthcare context map. This map then illuminates how communications might be shared or implemented across the entire system.

Message Map

A message map is the basic framework used in creating compelling, relevant, and engaging messages for various healthcare audience segments (patient, caregiver, internal

stakeholder). A message map can also serve as an organizational alignment tool to ensure message consistency.
These maps are excellent for designing and implementing
messages across multiple stakeholders.

Needs Map

A Needs Map is generally intended to help map the needs of
various stakeholders and identify ways to impact stakeholders in a productive manner. There are many needs at play
within a given encounter, and all stakeholders have primary
and secondary needs. A needs map focuses on "behavior
levers" that can impact behavior change. Primary needs
can be appreciation, acceptance, and approval. Secondary
needs might be admiration, pity, intelligence, or power—
these needs are often hidden desires that the stakeholder
wants to keep private.

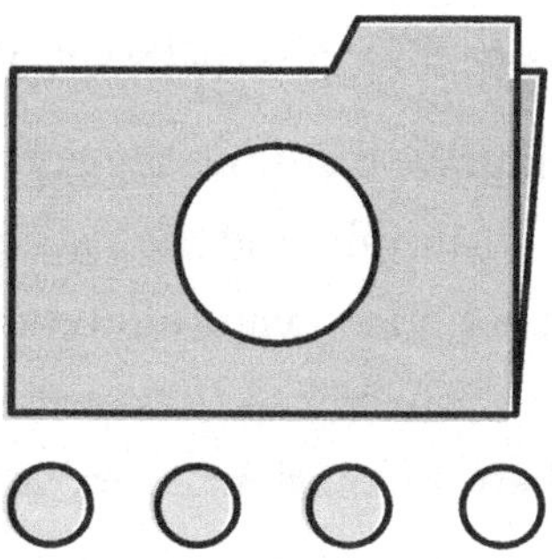

Asset Map

Asset mapping is a way of understanding the strengths and resources of a department, cohort, or the community at large. It's an excellent way to uncover potential solution designs. Once stakeholder strengths and resources are illuminated and depicted in a map, healthcare strategists and designers can more easily think about how to leverage the various assets to address organizational or community needs and improve health and well-being.

The use of mapping tools and illustrations are extremely helpful when presenting our insights to clients and related stakeholders. Maps are even more valuable when we seek to leverage insights and findings into the marketing, communication (internal or external), and patient education programs we design and implement. As marketing and patient (and stakeholder) engagement professionals, we play an important role in a brand's success, and mapping is a crucial component. Every action we take is intended to empower the patient and improve their health, whether the client is a pharmaceutical company, hospital, or health network.

JOURNEY MAPPING: A FAVORITE IN HEALTHCARE

In journey mapping, we examine the entire customer journey to reveal their triumphs and their struggles throughout the process. This enhanced view allows us to better understand the patient's journey so that we can improve upon it and make it a better experience for everyone involved.

Over time, as outreach continues and programs that provide support and education are developed, the journey map becomes an increasingly valuable resource. It illuminates how we might interact with patients in a natural, personal way that demonstrates an understanding beyond what the patient expects from a researcher.

MAPPING THE JOURNEY OF THE PEDIATRIC URGENT CARE EXPERIENCE

Think about a parent taking their child to an urgent care center. There are a variety of factors that influence their experience and impact the value of their visit. Sometimes they have other kids with them, and long wait times are nearly impossible to withstand. They're worried about their child in an anxiety-inducing environment, with forms to complete and insurance cards to present.

This is where ethnography enables us to deliver the best solution possible. By embedding ourselves in the natural context of everyday life, we understand the journey a patient (or in this case, the parent) takes in urgent care, from onset of illness to the minute they walk through the front door, to the moment they're discharged back into the community.

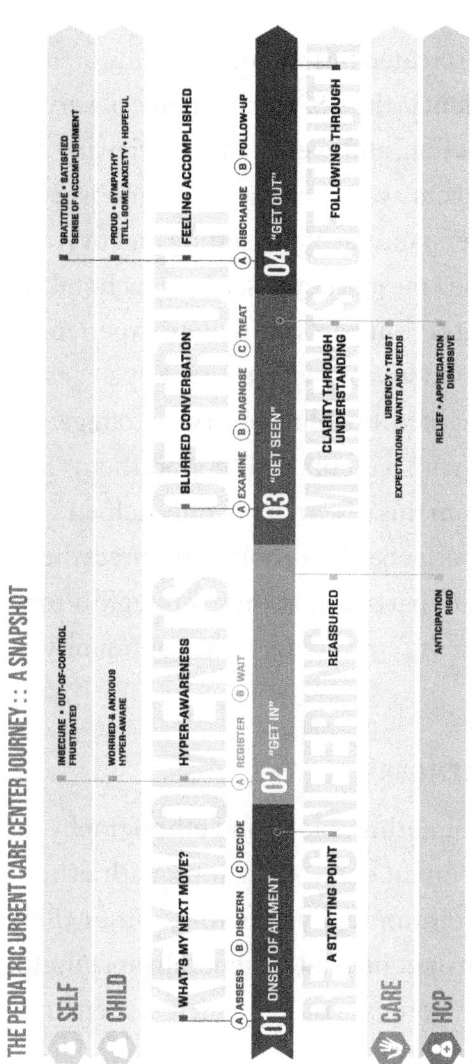

This four-phase journey map illustrates the various "actors" in the pediatric urgent care journey: *child*, *parent*, *healthcare professional*, and the intersection of these players with *care* delivery.

At LIFT, we created this map in our study of urgent care centers for a client in the US. We spent time observing behaviors, communication, and events. By interviewing and observing the key players, we supplemented our observations with a better understanding of the setting and overall experience. We examined the journey to see how each stakeholder's reality in urgent care impacts the patient experience from both a functional and sensory perspective. Key stages in the journey were highlighted, enabling us to see strategic opportunities to connect with patients and support them. The insight we gleaned from this research not only helped us improve the patient experience, it also helped us direct the urgent care's marketing department in their strategic efforts to market their services to consumers in the community.

THE CHALLENGERS

The path for anthropology and ethnography in healthcare has not been an easy one. Along with other qualitative methods, ethnography explains, rather than measures. We offer insight instead of generalizable findings, and we generate hypotheses rather than test them. It's qualitative, not quantitative.

Often, we find that healthcare executives are narrowly focused on quantitative data, overlooking the value of qualitative insight. Skeptics doubt that qualitative research provides the value to healthcare that quantitative data can provide. Admittedly, it's difficult to evaluate ethnographical evidence with a standardized set of criteria. Ethnography done well, however, delivers thematic context and important data that will support the value of such interviews and observations and complement the quantitative data that many healthcare strategists crave. The generalizability of our data is also a debated topic, with supporters believing that qualitative research requires its own set of criteria to qualify as generalizable.

Our approach is about innovation and quality design—both provide long-term value rather than immediate economic or financial benefits. In every industry, money is a powerful force that sometimes forsakes quality for quantity. Ethnography *is* expensive and labor-intensive. Can we place a value, though, on an improved understanding of the patient? What is the value of customer insight? Our answers lie in how we leverage this knowledge to impact the financial and economic performance of our brands.

EVERYONE WINS

In 2017, the Food and Drug Administration held a public meeting for psoriasis patients and their caregivers. They were hoping to gain insight into the effects of the disease and wanted to open a discussion about current therapy options. Many of the most important stakeholders were present. In addition to patients and caregivers, clinicians and researchers attended and took the opportunity to hear, firsthand, how psoriasis impacted the daily life of those who were affected by it.

Such an interactive approach was a very fresh first step toward better understanding and hearing the patient's voice. This initiative was part of the FDA's recent commitment to actively seek out patient perspectives about their condition and available therapies.

The focus of the meeting was on the symptoms of psoriasis and the impact of the disease, but no topic was off-limits. Patients spoke about the emotional toll of living with daily pain and active flare-ups, from the embarrassment and social discrimination, to how the disease limits an active lifestyle. Psoriasis is hereditary, so patients and family members shared the impact the disease has had on multiple generations.

In this groundbreaking meeting, patients discussed the routes of administration for their prescription and non-prescription medicines, the success or failure of various experimental therapies, and their struggle for clarity from providers and the hospitals and health networks that support them. Participants also explored pediatric psoriasis, a subcategory of which clinicians and researchers know very little. The spectrum of discussion and the exchange of knowledge made this a valuable human research experiment in a public space.

For the pharmaceutical companies and healthcare providers in attendance, the information shared in events like this is extremely valuable. As their marketing agency, we can take this knowledge and follow it up with our own ethnographic study to support patient outreach, education, and advocacy. We can also use it for regulatory packaging or a product launch. From here, we can develop clinical training around the biopsychosocial effects of psoriasis to help clinical professionals, caregivers, and patients understand and learn how to manage the various aspects of their condition beyond their technical diagnosis. We can create educational materials, build a website that offers online counseling, or a registry of resources like articles, support groups, and small research projects for psoriasis patients struggling with the emotional impact of their disease.

With a commitment to ethnography and patient centricity, we can reshape a healthcare brand's commercial and marketing approach, enabling our clients to demonstrate that they understand their patients with more impactful communication and patient education.

THE HEART OF IT ALL

The value of ethnography in healthcare is obvious. It uncovers insight into the lived experience of patients we care for and care about. With it, the patient's voice is heard, and their experience is examined as if it matters—because it does. Ultimately, this empowers patients to make important decisions and take an active role in their course of treatment. These are changes in patient mindset and behavior that will have a sustainable impact on the entire system.

Anthropology enables collaboration between the patient and the healthcare solution we represent. The patient is the expert who the rest of us rely on for insight and awareness. They are the heart of our business, and the reason we have a purpose.

— CHAPTER 4 —

DESIGN THINKING

Design thinking uses creative activities to foster collaboration and solve problems in human-centered ways. Design thinking leads to creative confidence. Creative confidence is the belief that everyone is creative, and that creativity isn't the ability to draw or compose or sculpt, but a way of understanding the world.

DAVID KELLEY, FOUNDER OF IDEO

If you conduct a quick search on "design thinking," you'll most likely read discussions about prototyping and collaborating, and you'll find success stories about how businesses and global nonprofits utilize design for instrumental change. You probably won't see a lot about the use of design thinking in healthcare, but this is changing.

As with ethnography, the patient and virtually any stakeholder in the healthcare transaction is the expert in design thinking. Patient involvement is more than ideal—it's essential. We can think of it as a fancy name for problem-solving and brainstorming, but it deserves any bit of grandeur we assign it. Anthropology in combination with design thinking is the perfect solution for a patient-centered approach in healthcare marketing and design strategy.

WHAT IS DESIGN THINKING?

Design thinking is not about the fragmental use of ads, logos, or social media. It doesn't cultivate gimmicky marketing. Rather, it's about identifying how a brand interacts with a target audience and how it empowers them. Simply stated, design thinking is innovative problem-solving that focuses on the value a solution will provide all stakeholders. In healthcare, it requires a deep understanding of the human condition—which is why it pairs well with ethnography.

Design thinking is comprehensive, yet detailed. It enables us to understand the relationship between many elements in a process, while recognizing opportunities to improve them. Most importantly, it directs us to observe the individual as they relate to the whole. Overall, design thinking allows companies to differentiate themselves from their competition—and those who employ the tools and protocols of design will typically have an advantage.

In healthcare, design thinking picks up where ethnography leaves off while still utilizing empathy throughout the process. Everything we learn about the patient's reality through ethnographic research methods is used in design thinking to build better solutions and improve how we both interact and communicate with that patient.

With design thinking, the more stakeholders involved, the better, and solutions are limitless. The results of design thinking can take many different forms. They can identify tools to help parents better understand how to adhere to prescribed treatments for their child, provide checklists for effective communication between clinician and patient during an urgent care visit, and facilitate clinical trial recruitment and retention best practices. These results can also influence educational materials that help patients navigate a particular illness and empower them to make healthier life choices. There is a multitude of uses for design thinking—the list could go on and on. The essential idea behind design is to leverage inputs from multiple stakeholders and look at multiple ways to solve problems.

At LIFT, the protocols of design thinking have been successfully leveraged to iteratively improve upon many healthcare processes and experiences. When children visit the pediatric urgent care, we helped to improve the intake process and waiting room environment. In clinical trials, we developed educational materials for more efficient recruitment and retention of participants. We've also used design to inform service line strategies as well as capital campaigns for hospitals.

In pharma, we've conducted numerous immersions in order to understand the burden of disease and therapy in areas such as rheumatic diseases, pediatric care transition, bipolar disorder, and others—all intended to inform patient-first branding, marketing, and stakeholder-education strategies. For a women's health service, we coordinated the interactions amongst the various healthcare providers, and we created school-based healthcare programming for children eligible for Medicaid.

Overall, we use design thinking to create more patient-focused experiences while simultaneously promoting the brand and its longevity. As a result, the healthcare providers we work with have healthier, happier patients and successful products that serve communities to the best of their ability.

As we design experiences, our goal is to help both patients and healthcare providers move through a healthcare encounter in a way that empowers patients to make their own decisions about therapies and treatments. We ask the important questions: What resources might the healthcare provider need to assist them in educating the patient? What barriers stand in the way of the patient absorbing this knowledge and increasing their competency? What does a typical day look like for a patient and their family? When does the patient feel most vulnerable? What kind of social pressures do they experience?

Ethnography provides us perspective. Design thinking gives us a process for creatively addressing strategic imperatives. Understanding the potential barriers in our design allows us to account for pitfalls and guide the patient closer to complete accountability.

THE PHASES OF DESIGN THINKING

In design thinking, we connect with those who will benefit from potential design solutions, and we explore our ideas in a collaborative environment. We then test the most promising designs for efficacy—keeping an open mind for the need to improve or iterate on an envisioned solution.

It's important to note that design is not a linear process. It's intended to be iterative and cyclical. Because of this, returning to a previous phase in an effort to redefine a failed prototype is not uncommon. Not until a prototype is tested and retested do we truly understand how it supports our objective and serves the patient. Prototypes can be nothing more than an embodied idea—a clear picture of an idea that serves as a foundation.

Let's look at these phases in more detail to understand how design thinking works.

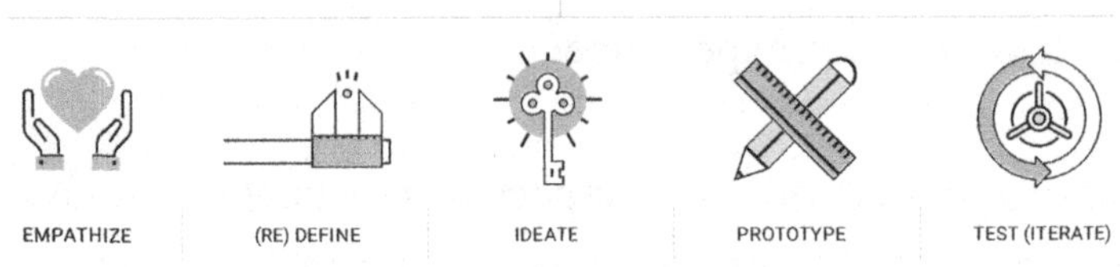

EMPATHIZE

The first phase of design thinking is dependent upon ethnography to gain a clear understanding of the stakeholders involved. In this stage, we determine what people think, feel, say, and believe.

During the empathize stage, we talk to a wide range of patients and related stakeholders (family, caregivers, clinical staff, and more) to understand their beliefs about the condition or area of focus and to observe their routine. We find out what motivates or discourages the patient about their disease and related therapy so we can understand the cultural and social context. During one project at LIFT, for example, we helped older pediatric patients living with juvenile idiopathic arthritis (JIA) transition from pediatric care to adult care. This is a stressful time for the patient, their parents, and even for their pediatrician who has cared for the patient for years. JIA is a lifelong disease, and understanding all the challenges a high school student living with JIA faces was an extensive process. Not only are they becoming adults, but they are becoming adult *patients*. They're leaving their pediatrician for a new doctor (usually an adult rheumatologist) in addition to graduating from high school, possibly entering college, and facing social and sexual maturity.

In this phase, it was important for us to understand the reality for both the patient and their parents so that we could improve these transitions. We examined ways we could facilitate a better exchange of information between patient and physician, patient and parent, parent and physician, and physician and physician. How could we stress the importance of treatment adherence in a way that resonated with the patient? Could we help the patient navigate their new social narrative, especially as it pertained to their condition? Was there a role the pediatrician could play in facilitating a smooth transition to adult care? How can we empower parents to let go? These were the types of questions we asked ourselves during this phase. The goal was to gather enough observations to truly understand the entire stakeholder perspective.

DEFINE

The define phase is when we combine our research results and analyze our opportunities to create better outcomes. This is also when we examine each intersection between patient and stakeholder—whether caregiver, physician, or friend.

In our JIA project, we noticed that many parents had the tendency to overcompensate for their child's condition by doing things for them that the child should learn to do for themselves. They struggled to reconcile their overwhelming sense of obligation with the pending loss of control, inadvertently making for a more challenging transition into adulthood for the patient. Many of the patients see their parents as an emotional and social hindrance. Not only do they struggle with articulating their frustration to their parents, but social pressures weigh them down, causing them to feel lost and overwhelmed. They want to express freedom from both their parents and their disease.

Their particular situation was well-defined, offering many opportunities to facilitate a better outcome for the patient, their parents, and their relationship. Once we define the areas in which we can focus our solutions, we ideate.

IDEATE

Ideation is brainstorming on steroids. This is the phase when we convene to think of creative and strategically sound solutions that address the unmet patient needs identified in Define.

We want to allow ourselves complete freedom during ideation. No idea goes unlisted, and no judgments are passed. It's quantity over quality. This is our chance to articulate our vision and pull our informed thoughts together. It's also when we build on the good ideas and eliminate the weak. We polish the best ideas and move them on to the Prototype phase.

After we uncovered the unmet needs of our JIA patients, we explored ways we could openly acknowledge the frustrations of both patient and parent, while also offering healthier care and disease management. We brainstormed tools and experiences that would bring the patient and parent to a common place of understanding and empowerment. We cultivated several ideas, then moved into the prototype phase for further testing and refinement.

PROTOTYPE

The Prototype phase is where we make our ideas and concepts tactile. We may combine two or three smaller ideas to create a solution, or we may have one great idea.

The Prototype phase is about understanding what works and what doesn't work. Some solutions that seem perfect are infeasible to implement. It's worth our time, however, to fight for the ideas that have the greatest impact. This is also when we begin testing the proposed solutions that made it this far in the design thinking process. Feedback is important, and the best solutions always include real patients.

For our JIA patients, we crafted educational tools for the

various stakeholders that allowed them to embark on a journey toward mutual understanding. We started a conversation in which everyone could feel heard, allowing progress to be made in the patient's care and disease management. We created a set of journey maps for the patient and parent, highlighting our opportunities to learn more. The end result was a set of learning and trivia cards intended to elicit conversation between patient and parent that was grounded in mutual understanding and growth.

TESTING THE PROTOTYPE

The actual Test phase is when we bring one solution to the various stakeholders involved and gather their feedback. We ask them—and ourselves—if the solution addresses the needs, and whether it improves the way they think or feel. Is the patient able to connect with their healthcare provider and caregivers easier, and will this make a positive impact on education and empowerment?

The objective of this testing and refining phase is to verify that our design achieves our intended goals. We ask ourselves and program participants additional questions to triple-check that our design is a strong solution with a meaningful impact on the patient experience and their overall treatment.

When we tested our first prototype for our JIA patients, we

learned that the physician had a role in this new conversation. Some of the content included in the trivia cards was clinically connected to the care experience. In observing patient and parent interaction with the cards, we realized that a facilitator with a clinical perspective could increase the value of the discussion to all involved. We added a step in the design that included the healthcare provider introducing the patient and parent to the cards while in a clinical setting. This simple step eased anxiety about the transition from pediatric to adult care for both the patient and the parent, assuring them that all parties would be involved in the discussion *and* that tools were available to help them with the transition.

This typical process of design, test, and refine is crucial to understanding the potential of a proposed solution. For our JIA study, we went through several test and refine cycles (and continue to do so) in order to create a truly impactful resource.

Once there's a tested and verified solution design, it's time to implement.

IMPLEMENT

This phase is where we see our efforts unfold to a wider audience. This is when the finalized solution is built—when our design finally comes to life.

Implement is an important phase of design thinking because it's the reason why we engage in design thinking in the first place. It's why we empathize with patients and brainstorm ideas, and then test, and retest. Although some designs fail and others succeed, after our building and rebuilding—we find a solution that makes us proud and improves the lives of each patient.

There's an awesome saying by esteemed design expert, Diego Rodriguez: "Prototype as if you are right. Listen as if you are wrong." It's popular because it's true. Once we have a strong prototype to test with stakeholders, we build it with conviction. The test phase is when we show our humility, absorb feedback, and either shape it into a new prototype or move forward with implementation. Sometimes, we may even scrap the idea completely. Because this multidisciplinary approach impacts everyone, it's important to keep an open mind. We can learn valuable insights from both our stakeholders and other team members.

4 ORDERS OF DESIGN

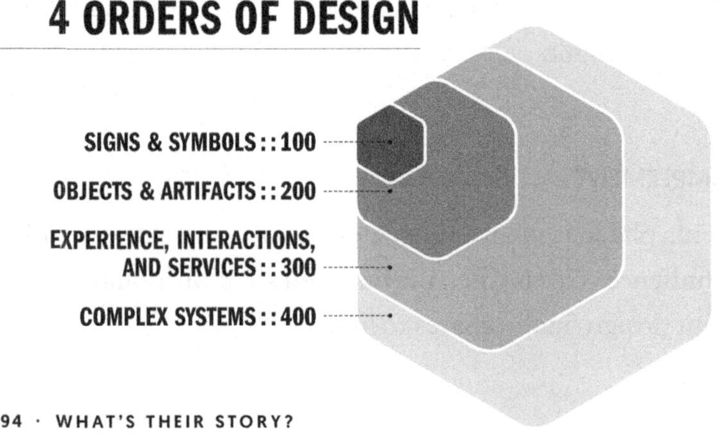

RICHARD BUCHANAN'S FOUR ORDERS OF DESIGN

At LIFT, we honor the esteemed design theorist Richard Buchanan's Four Orders of Design. We use it as a framework in designing brands, marketing strategies, and developing educational materials that support the patient experience:

1. Signs and Symbols: This is the work of graphic and communication designers. Signs and symbols give an intentional voice to our organization, representing our values and beliefs and enabling us to impact the behavior of others. In our work with the JIA patients, the words, illustrations, photographs, and graphs were the symbols we used to express the concepts.

2. Objects and Artifacts: These are the results of prototype design. In marketing, artifacts can be physical or digital—medical devices and medications are artifacts, as are brochures, websites, and even trivia cards. We use objects and artifacts, in addition to signs and symbols, to empower consumer behavior.

3. Experience, Interactions, and Services: As healthcare marketers, we ask ourselves how the interactions and services of our brands impact the patient experience. This is when we identify opportunities for improvement and any gaps in the system. Our JIA trivia cards created a conversation and empowered an experience—interacting with these cards is an experience.

4. Complex Systems: The last order refers to almost any system. The global healthcare system is an enormous and complex system—primary care, as a subsystem of the larger healthcare landscape, also shares complexity. The learning and trivia cards in our JIA work are intended to encourage conversations that impact not only the pediatric patients, their parents, and their healthcare providers, but also the success of the larger, more complex system of healthcare.

The beauty of design thinking is that it's open-ended and vulnerable. There are many witnesses to our successes and failures, and that's okay—the best solutions often emerge from failed designs.

Design thinking can feel like we're trying to cage a wild animal. If we do it right, it *should* feel free and unruly. These phases simply ensure what eventually becomes innate for all design thinkers in healthcare—the patient and all related stakeholders are the experts. Our best solutions always come from insights grounded in each stakeholder's personal perspective and experience.

WHY DO WE USE DESIGN THINKING?

Design thinking is difficult. Because it's a nonlinear process, designers must be patient, adaptive, and eager to learn. Many find it frustrating, especially those who want quick solutions and a consistent process. The question stands: What's the benefit of such a challenging process?

We understand that design thinking is a human-centered approach, but there are other reasons why it's an ideal process for creating valuable solutions in the healthcare world. Innovation, behind human centricity, is a leading tenet of design thinking. We see this in the ideation phase as we unleash our creativity and focus on quantity over quality. In an otherwise structured process, ideation allows us to let our imaginations take us where we need to go in the design cycle.

The list of possible healthcare stakeholders who have both something to gain *and* something to offer in the design thinking process is nearly endless. This is not a system for only marketers or branding professionals. In fact, design thinking provides a place for everyone to come together. How often does a brand executive intersect with scientists at a pharmaceutical company, an operations executive intersect with marketing strategists in a hospital, or a trialist converse with marketers? Design facilitates such collisions and fuels thinking across a diverse swath of stakeholders. It's rare to have a sanctioned environment for all departments to gather and explore solutions. That's the beauty of design.

Design thinking leverages a wide range of expertise, both inside and outside an organization. This involvement from multiple stakeholders contributes to innovation and patient centricity. It unites everyone in a shared language and common goal—healthcare providers, clinical staff, medical educators, commercial and clinical marketers, and, most importantly, patients and their caregivers.

CHAPTER 5

WHAT WE CAN LEARN FROM PUBLIC HEALTH AND PALLIATIVE CARE

The definitive factors in determining whether someone is in good health extend significantly beyond access to care, and include the conditions in their life and the conditions of their neighborhoods and communities.

JOHN AUERBACH, ASSOCIATE DIRECTOR FOR POLICY AT CENTERS FOR DISEASE CONTROL AND PREVENTION

Public health is a blending of healthcare and government initiatives that's not often fully understood by the people it serves. It has a global reach, protecting and improving the health of smaller communities, which each feed into larger communities and comprise the general masses. Public health is our local health departments, the Food and Drug Administration, the Centers for Disease Control and Prevention, the National Institutes of Health, and a myriad of other organizations that work toward the public's welfare. Whether it's a nationwide food recall, HIV education for teens, diabetes education in poor communities, or a global pandemic—public health researches, educates, and informs. Ultimately, public health has our back.

Many patients and consumers recognize public health, but few truly understand it. The same can be said about palliative care. Most think of hospice and end-of-life treatment, but palliative care extends far beyond end-of-life treatment. Palliative care and public health have similar goals, yet their strongest connection is their patient philosophy. At the heart of both public health and palliative care is the patient and a desire to lessen suffering and empower a better quality of life.

It's easy for contemporary healthcare companies to feel like pioneers in patient centricity, but public health and palliative care have roots that reach back as far as 1916. This was when John Hopkins University opened the first school of public health with money from a Rockefeller Foundation grant. Later, in 1963, a woman named Dame Cicely Saunders spoke at Yale University and introduced the idea of providing specialized care to the dying. It could be said that Dame Saunders was a kind of public health advocate in Great Britain. She trained as a nurse, then as a social worker. She's noted for her work in terminal care research and her role in the birth of the hospice movement—subsequently starting the first hospice and paving the way for the discovery and refinement of the palliative care movement.

Because of these early pioneers in the biopsychosocial model, patient-centeredness has evolved into what it is today. Their efforts have allowed us to leverage what they know and expand it to better identify the importance of patient centricity in today's world. By placing the patient at the center of the conversation, both public health and palliative care are better able to positively affect the communities in which they serve.

PUBLIC HEALTH

Public health has five core disciplines: behavioral science and health education, biostatistics, environmental health, epidemiology, and health services administration.

With behavioral science and health education as a core discipline, it's easy to see how public health draws on the work of Balint and neatly intersects with efforts in patient education, service design, treatment outreach, and drug development. Patient behavior and education are also the primary areas in which all healthcare marketers have an impact. Public health recognizes that understanding the patient's reality is paramount to empowering the patient in their own health and well-being. It's equally important in building a better treatment experience for healthier outcomes.

Public health is more than just disease prevention and community outreach, it's human and cultural understanding. It's also community and patient empowerment that's intended to prolong life, promote good health and well-being, and empower behaviors through outreach and education. Not only has the public health system for solving healthcare issues proven it works over an extended period of time, but their solutions both educate *and* empower patients.

Education is at the core of public health outreach, from marketing aimed at patients with particular illnesses to programs focused on the promotion of a healthy lifestyle. Their motivation is to protect individuals, their communities, and our entire population—whether it's rescuing a suburban neighborhood in Wylie, Texas from disease, or shielding the entire United States from a nationwide outbreak. One of the best aspects of public health is that their outreach extends not only to patients, but to their support network. These are the stakeholders in a healthcare transaction. They are the patients, the clinical professionals, the government agencies, and the caregivers who often need just as much support as the patients themselves. Success, at the patient level, means shared success for entire communities.

In recent years we've seen fantastic examples of how public health can integrate with primary care. Public health is often the first and occasionally the only stop in healthcare for many. This remarkable integration offers opportunities for improved quality of care and lower overall health costs. This type of collaboration not only expands the reach of public health initiatives, but it illuminates how public health intersects with a patient-centered philosophy.

When the Connecticut Department of Public Health (CDPH) collaborated with primary healthcare organizations, their aim was to educate asthma sufferers about their condition and reduce emergency room visits. They established Putting on AIRS, or Asthma Indoor Risk Strategies, a statewide, in-home visitation program that educates patients and their families about indoor asthma triggers. Through this program, nurses obtain referrals and then visit the homes of asthma patients. They conduct in-home assessments and develop a personalized action plan to reduce or eliminate the sources of the patient's triggers.

The program was a success. At onset, only 20 percent of program participants met the criteria for well-controlled asthma, while 16 percent met the criteria for not-well-controlled asthma, and a clear majority of 64 percent met the criteria for very poorly controlled asthma. After just six months of Putting on AIRS, the majority turned into the minority with just 13 percent of participants meeting the criteria for very poorly controlled asthma. Additionally, the number of asthma-related, unscheduled acute care visits decreased by 87 percent, saving approximately $26,720 per one hundred patients. Participants reported a reduction in their rescue inhaler use by 74 percent, and the number of days missed at work or school also decreased significantly by 82 percent.

The Putting on AIRS program is a good example of a public health initiative that uses the patient's reality as a cornerstone of strategy. It also demonstrates the value of putting the patient and their lived reality first. Their target audience *and* ours is the patient, and engagement strategies leveraging the public health philosophy have shown us that patient-centered care can often deliver the best solution.

PALLIATIVE CARE

Palliative care is a concept that goes hand in hand with the goals of public health. The health of every community, big and small, comprises the health of the nation in public healthcare. Their treatment must be efficient and effective. Even still, as we've learned from Putting on AIRS, the best treatment plan starts with the patient's story. Palliative care has a more focused client base with a bigger, multidisciplinary team working toward their patient's well-being. But patient understanding, efficiency, and treatment effectiveness are just as important in palliative care as in public health.

Those who work in palliative care strive to understand the patient and the family members in their own environments. All stakeholders face problems with a patient's illness—especially in a life-threatening illness—and palliative care works toward improving the quality of life for all involved. Palliative care is known for its significant impact on the patient and their support system. With symptoms controlled, stress for both the patient and family is also controlled. Additionally, competency improves when stakeholders are empowered, competent, and feel understood.

This is no easy task, but palliative care professionals have an extensive background in a variety of disciplines. From primary care physicians and long-term care staff to hospice workers and nurse practitioners, they start by finding ways to prevent and relieve suffering for their patients by first understanding their story. In addition to coordinating an often complex medical journey, palliative care professionals use environmental assessments and in-home interviewing to absorb everything about the patient and their caregivers. By doing this, they can offer the best path forward—both medically and emotionally.

Pain relief, mental illness, family dynamics, home care, and spiritual concerns all fall under the realm of palliative care. True relief for chronic illness can only come when we consider everything that impacts a patient. Every patient and stakeholder is unique, with different experiences and individual circumstances. No two patients are alike. Because of this, palliative care allows us to see the patient in their unique environment to determine and address true stakeholder needs.

PALLIATIVE CARE HITS HOME

The reality is that most of us will work with palliative care at some point in our lives. I have my own experience with palliative care, and my family has benefitted from its tools and interventions.

At eighty, my mother suffered from severe arthritis. She was ornery and independent, but she lost that independence when she became addicted to opioids—the solution she was prescribed for her chronic pain. Like many elderly patients across the country, her primary care doctors and pain medicine clinics failed her. Beyond their prescriptions, they offered her no personal support. As she struggled more and more with her life situation and her "prescribed" addiction, we children found ourselves placing her in an assisted living facility. In addition to the failure of the healthcare system (we all know about the opioid epidemic and how it has traumatized America), her assisted living facility failed her, too. Not only was there lack of attention to my mother's needs, but staff members were diverting opioids for street use. It was a complete mess.

Our entire family struggled to find the best treatment partners and plan for her. As her children, we worked hard to intervene and understand her needs by calling and visiting her, asking her questions, and trying to get involved with her care system. As an addict surrounded by caregivers who were themselves addicts, we were easily manipulated. This made the problems difficult to identify. Some things were clear: She was not compliant with her medications, her pain doctors were blind to her actual needs, and she lacked proper care in her living facility.

My mother was falling through the cracks in the healthcare system, and other than family members, no one was noticing—whether that was her doctors or one of her caregivers. After a two-year battle with opioid addiction and her failing health, hospice became involved in her treatment. They interviewed all the stakeholders in my mother's situation, starting with us children. They placed my siblings and me in the middle of the transaction, pushing those who previously showed no interest in a tailored treatment plan to the outside. Palliative care came to my mother's aid—and ours.

With palliative care professionals involved, we learned techniques to better manage our mom's needs. Not only did we learn strategies that we could use to help our mother, but we were given valuable tools that we could use to help ourselves. We learned how to approach and improve our relationship with everyone involved in the process. This included our relationship with our mother, our relationship with each other, and our relationship with the caregivers we were having a difficult time trusting. We were provided with educational materials, guidance, and resources that helped us understand our rights and responsibilities in caring for an elderly woman suffering from pain.

My mother never fully overcame her addiction, but her physical, mental, and emotional health did improve slightly with the help of palliative care. We saw her living facility in a different light, too. We came to the understanding that they offered her only what they could—and it simply wasn't enough for our mom. Add to that the assisted living facility had a less than quality staff, and we had our hands full.

Soon after palliative care intervened, we relocated mom to the home of my sister. Although she continued to battle opioid addiction, she was under the care of healthcare providers who we could trust and who helped us understand the importance of comfort. We tried tapering her off the opioids, but the damage was done. Even though we had a very useful set of tools, which we gained through palliative care, we lost her not long after.

DIFFERENT, BUT THE SAME

They may be two different concepts, but public health and

palliative care share important similarities from which the rest of the healthcare system can learn.

First, they're unique because they embed themselves in a community to find the best care-delivery strategies available. This is how they improve a patient's quality of life. The best tool they have available to them is their ability to see the full picture—they understand how the mental, physical, social, and spiritual aspects work together to create the whole patient. Their mission is as much about improving overall well-being as it is improving health.

Public health and palliative care also both employ empathy to see healthcare through their patient's point of view—this is how they achieve their goals. Using empathy means knowing a patient's story *and* understanding how these details make all the difference in the treatment each patient receives. They also determine the level of each patient's own competence and accountability.

These models would achieve only half the level of success, however, if education was not at the forefront of their platforms. Education is the key to empowerment—and empowerment leads to patient accountability and healthier outcomes. This is how marketers improve the healthcare process, one patient story at a time.

As times and strategies change, so must the models we

use as examples. This is how public health and palliative care show us the path toward empathic patient care and treatment, and a better overall healthcare system. They work toward solving the entire problem rather than just the physical disease.

Our goal should be to engage and empower patients. This requires a mindset shift based on empathy and patient centricity, which is the foundation of a healthcare marketing approach based on the biopsychosocial model. While the solution is not complete without anthropology and design thinking, understanding a better method—and a better mindset—is the first step. Once we embrace a patient-centric approach, we become more valuable stakeholders in the discussion that answers the ultimate question: How do we improve healthcare?

CHAPTER 6

CHAMPIONING THE PATIENT

Patient understanding is just as important as science, technology, and molecules. The biopsychosocial model of healthcare illuminates how impactful human understanding is to the continued evolution of healthcare as a business.

MATT BRADLEY, HEALTHCARE ANTHROPOLOGIST AT LIFT

A stronger platform of patient centricity is emerging in healthcare, thanks in part to our transition from a biomedical model to biopsychosocial one. We see patients differently now. In fact, we see health and well-being differently now, too. Diseases are no longer isolated to their physical manifestations. Within every patient suffering from an illness lies the psychological and sociological impact of their disease—an undeniable fact. This realization not only provides significant advantage to each patient, but it also provides valuable insight for our brands and businesses.

From Enid Balint and Dame Cicely Saunders to George Engel, these early innovators of patient centricity paved the way for this change. They were few, but their voices and theories revolutionized healthcare, making it possible for others to take the baton and advocate for a new perspective.

As renowned design theorist Richard Buchanan might say, creating a truly patient-centered system of care is a "wicked design problem" because it's difficult to solve. It's an important step in the evolution of healthcare that requires time, resources, and the right mindset for progress. I believe we're on our way to a healthcare industry that fully champions the patient voice across every domain of strategy and care. I think of this transformative journey we're on within the context of the innovation adoption curve discussed by Everett Rogers and his colleagues in 1957.

Rogers' renowned book, *Diffusion of Innovations*, is one of the oldest discussions of social science theory. In his book, Rogers explains his theory of innovation adoption, illustrating that new concepts and ideas gain momentum and diffuse throughout a social system over time. The same can be said for the evolution of patient centricity.

ROGER'S INNOVATION ADOPTION CURVE

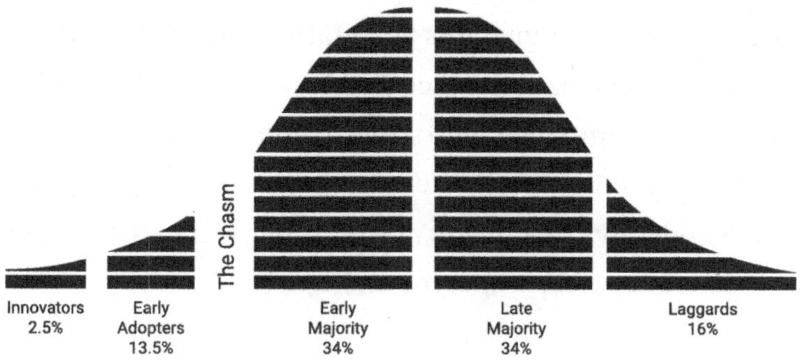

The path we've traveled over the past fifty years is a perfect example of how an industry adopts new ideas to evolve. The supporters, explorers, and practitioners of patient centricity have gained significant momentum in the past seven years, offering proof that this innovation is becoming mainstream. Better systems of care grounded in the patient's perspective are now not only accepted, but embraced.

Rogers tells us that the majority finds most innovations in the early stages risky. To mitigate feelings of uncertainty, likeminded people look for others who agree with them as the innovation matures. According to Rogers' construct, these pioneers are the innovators and early adaptors who comprise only a small percentage of the larger population of people who could benefit from the innovation.

If Enid Balint and George Engel are the innovators of patient centricity, then today's companies and health-care providers who consider themselves patient-focused, regardless of their specific place in the market, are the early adopters. This list includes hospitals and health networks that rely on the patient voice in their care. It also includes life science companies who strive to understand the patient experience more clearly. We're making significant progress in our collective healthcare priorities by putting the patient first to create more impactful therapies.

CROSSING THE CHASM

As an industry, we're on the brink of crossing the chasm into a new paradigm that Rogers calls "the early majority." We have theories and models to guide our way. Our examples are Enid Balint, George Engle, Dame Cicely Saunders, and our collective work over the last ten years. Through these examples, we see what the entire industry is capable of becoming. Crossing that chasm is symbolic of the rebirth of how we market—how we engage with, educate, and empower the users of our brands and thereby empower our brands for success.

Anthropology and design thinking are the most important tools we have as contemporary healthcare strategists and marketers. We have the opportunity to make the patient experience everyone's responsibility, setting the stage for an era of healthcare that puts the patient's voice above all else.

When a solution works, everyone wants to learn more. If a

pharmaceutical company designs a way to make patients more competent, healthcare providers want to know how they can use this method in their own approach. The discussion about patient centricity, anthropology, and design thinking includes more members of the healthcare industry (and more stakeholders in the healthcare transaction) every day, and efforts are becoming increasingly collaborative.

THE EVOLUTION OF PATIENT CENTRICITY

Our one consistency, no matter the theory or strategic approach we embrace, is the patient. Technology improves, science evolves, and values change, but the patient will always remain the most important (and complex) element in the healthcare conversation. Understanding them is as paramount as it is complicated—and a task we as anthropologists and designers are up to.

Patient centricity has more meaning today than it did in Balint's time. It used to mean asking the patient *any* question beyond the status of their physical health. Basic questions that inquired about a patient's marital status, number of children, or the health of their parents qualified as a patient-centered approach. Drawing inspiration from the pioneers of ethnography like Malinowski and Mead, we now have the tools and resources to immerse ourselves into the patient's reality and observe them and ask questions that elicit deeper responses. When applied correctly, these tools provide us with the ability to uncover human-centered insight into the complex realities of the stakeholder's lived experience, which provides a rock-solid foundation for design.

HOW TO INFLUENCE CHANGE AND FOSTER ACCOUNTABILITY

We know that our brands improve with the patient's perspective, and that the information they provide is invaluable for effective communication and future research. We also know that our solutions are more impactful *and* profitable when we use ethnography and design thinking to inform our strategies. Whether every hospital, healthcare network, health practitioner, or industry executive truly understands the potential of patient centricity is irrelevant because we are crossing that chasm—regardless of the soon-to-be minority.

Our answer to a better healthcare system is less elusive than we may have thought, and it's grounded in a better understanding of the patient and his or her lived reality. A better healthcare system directly benefits the patient, and a competent and accountable patient benefits the overall healthcare system. We know that competent patients can be born from brands that engage the patient and educate them in their own care. We also know that relevant messaging is how we cultivate the kind of competency that fuels accountability.

This is where understanding heuristics is important. Heuristics is an approach to problem-solving, learning, and discovery that enables people to learn individually and in their own time. Patients and caregivers, for example, make their own decisions about treatment based on individual, cultural, and community values. The best healthcare brands are becoming choice architects, prompting and persuading patients toward a particular decision by creating an environment favorable to that decision. Essentially, with ethnography and design thinking, we have the power to positively inform how we influence patient decisions. We don't force outcomes, and we cannot control the will of a patient. We can, however, lead a patient toward a healthier decision that benefits everyone.

The concept of choice architecture is ideal for a healthcare brand interested in elevating consumer competency to create a more accountable patient. Education is the first step in structuring the patient's choice. After they have an increased awareness of their options, the next step is to illuminate and clarify their situation, enabling the patient to see *why* a particular treatment plan is more beneficial than another. Finally, the brand must demonstrate the value of the treatment to incentivize the patient's choice. They guide and support patients throughout, earning trust with every positive and personally relevant interaction. Choice architecture and heuristics rely on ethnography and design thinking to bring to life a patient-centered approach.

It's important to note that awareness and guidance must be framed in the appropriate context. This is why the foundation of any patient engagement or marketing strategy that is embodied in education must first seek to understand the human truths at ground level if they are to succeed.

IT'S TIME

The more time we spend working in this amazing space, the more we recognize that healthcare must change—and will change. It's inevitable. We additionally recognize that, as marketing professionals, we must also change. We work in an industry and system in constant movement, adjusting and progressing before our eyes. The power to influence this change is within us, but we have to leverage smart tools to affect that change. And I believe those important tools are anthropology and design.

Our profession is unique. It's easy for anyone to show up and clock out, but we have a responsibility in healthcare marketing to be innovators and lead the way to a more human-centered way of approaching patient interactions. Patients rely on their doctors as experts—we're experts, too. Patients rely on our messaging and guidance to help them make better choices. Whether you or they realize it or not, the words, pictures, values, and beliefs we espouse are inextricably linked to the experience a patient has with his or her own health. By allowing them to lead us, we're capable of developing solutions tailored to their needs and motivations.

It may be the first time that we truly understand the patients we serve. In knowing them better, we enable them to better understand themselves—and they enable us to better understand our brands. This is the key to building patient competency and accountability. The time is now for us to cross the chasm and embrace a better healthcare system. A rebirth in healthcare is happening regardless of how we react. Championing an anthropologist's mindset and the tools and protocols of design are table stakes if we want to be relevant as the strategists and marketers of tomorrow.

CHAPTER 7

A WORD ABOUT TECHNOLOGY

10 years after President Barack Obama signed a law to accelerate the digitization of medical records—with the federal government, so far, sinking $36 billion into the effort—America has little to show for its investment.

ERIKA FRY AND FRED SCHULTE (FORTUNE, 2019)

The US healthcare industry has invested billions on technology solutions in the past decade, but those solutions have largely failed to impact the cost or quality of care being delivered.

JEFF BECKER (FORRESTER.COM)

We all know that progress doesn't happen overnight. It's a slow, steady evolution of taking two steps forward and one step back. However, we culturally embrace certain forms of "progress" faster than others. Technology is one advancement that we're quick to incorporate into every aspect of our lives, but what does this cost us when we crown it the winning solution in patient care?

A few years back, I attended a two-day conference in San Francisco about technology in healthcare, hosted by Rock Health, a venture fund dedicated to digital health. By technology, I mean apps and related software for mobile devices. According to its website, Rock Health exists "to fund and support entrepreneurs working at the intersection of healthcare and technology." This particular conference was early in Rock Health's history (2014). The overarching conference narrative focused on (the now worn-out term) "disruption" and how apps will change the world. According to one speaker, the future "reality" of healthcare at the time was that of "the entire healthcare industry becoming an app." It seemed that everyone at the summit believed that innovation and (I hate to even use the word again) disruption grounded in technology was the key to ultimate transformation of the American (and even global) healthcare industry.

In one panel discussion called *Disrupting Regulated Industries*, Vivek Wadhwa, an American technology entrepreneur and academic, boldly stated that "A wave of disruption that no one understands, or no one can control is underway." He flatly stated that the entire "healthcare industry is becom-

ing an app" and that as an industry, "we have no security...
all the regulations protecting data are out the door." It was a
conference filled with bold claims and stunning predictions.
Wadhwa pontificated about the proliferation of human
genome testing, declaring, "In five years, we will be able
to sequence genome by just taking a glass someone has
drank out of, testing it, and then knowing everything about
them." Bold, right?

But the most compelling reflection Vivek shared was
around cardiology. While reflecting on a new app technology of the time period which offered EKG readings on a
mobile device (a tool something akin to the Kardia Mobile®
device that we see advertised all over TV these days), Vivek
stated that, "This entire concept of having to go to a car-
diologist for diagnosis has been upended already." That
seemed naïve to me, and not exactly accurate. What about
the human part—the patient or clinician? In response to a
video of Wadhwa saying these things, which was posted by
Rock Health, a viewer comment sums it up best:

> "This gentleman isn't any more visionary than some physi-
> cians and healthcare workers I work with; technology is a
> tool. But, "at this point of history," if anyone needs open heart
> surgery, he's going to need a team of human health workers
> in control of technology. And it isn't perfect, and as long as
> much of the disease states we are inflicted with, besides being
> genetically mediated, are socially propagated (e.g. obesity),

and are rooted to a degree in our stressful work environments and our life structures, and these won't be solved by apps soon, even though, we all hope that technology will help us..."

If you look at Rock's website, you can learn all about venture investing around healthcare and how great it looks through their lens—the lens of a cunning financial marketplace. In one Rock Health report "celebrating" the number of IPOs in 2019, you will read that digital health is "a robust sector receiving nearly one in ten venture dollars invested in the United States. In 2019, 359 US digital health start-ups raised $7.4B from 627 investors. Though six digital health companies entered the public markets in 2019, exits were a somewhat mixed bag, with M&A below trend at 112 deals across 2019." There's plenty of data celebrating the venture investing marketplace. Rightfully so. Rock is, after all, a financially focused organization seeking to connect early-stage businesses with investors looking for that next big financial success.

But I would ask: What is success for these tech companies? I realize that we can't go deep on a philosophical discussion of the intention or value of healthcare tech in this book, but I do think it's worth a short look. Is success for these early-stage businesses valuations that are likely as inflated as many of the Silicon Valley start-ups who have yet to turn a profit? Is success an IPO that makes the venture funds and entrepreneurs very rich? Is success to be viewed through a financial lens and in the short-term? Or should it be through the lens of a long-term, meaningful clinical and economic impact?

I believe that apps, technology, social media, and the like are a mile wide and an inch deep. In other words, it's gonna take a long, long time to find an app that impacts patient competency at scale across a wide swath of patients in a way that makes serious meaningful improvements in our healthcare system. I see this technology race as a financial one, rather than one that's grounded in a genuine understanding of the human condition. Sure, I believe there's obviously a focus on health, but I question the core intent of many of these tech applications when it comes to tackling the larger challenges associated with the human condition and humanity in healthcare.

While the proponents of technology claim that they start with the patient in mind, this is only true in that they're targeting users with a biomedical healthcare need. Their real focus is on a tech solution created in a type of echo chamber that will ultimately build perceived financial value in a business. They then sell the technology or capitalize on it like Uber or one of any of the hundreds of tech businesses still trying to generate a profit. The patient is interesting to them as long as they have a problem the company's tech solution can focus on. But the efficacy of their technological solutions is serving *their* purpose. Their ability to understand and improve patient health remains largely unproven. I challenge these innovators to dig in and truly champion the biopsychosocial model—those who do may just get it right someday.

I left the conference underwhelmed, but not discouraged. I saw an opportunity for people like myself—people who really want to improve healthcare and help create a better system—to step up and advocate for patient centricity in the face of advancing technology. I believe that change happens when we start inside the system, focusing on its purpose, complexity, and the people who constitute the reasons for the system in the first place.

LET'S HAVE A TALK—NOT A TEXT

There's value in health technology. Unfortunately, this value is lost when it distracts us from building genuine connections with the patients to whom we've devoted our careers. Sometimes we just need to talk, and in talking, we can share and learn from one another. I think a little more talking and a little less texting may be a positive thing.

Healthcare providers and pharmaceutical companies have been trying to leverage technology into their business strategies ever since Steve Jobs signed off on the first iPhone. Simultaneously, healthcare providers across the globe have struggled with how to champion the patient's reality ever since Enid Balint first compelled physicians to dig a little deeper into the patient's lived experience. It's complicated and, again, as Buchannan would say, it's a "wicked design problem"—one that anthropology and design can resolve as we seek to evolve and solve.

We all know that data is collected quicker and simpler when interacting with technology. We also understand that technology enables the measurement and analysis of patient data and even a patient's clinical journey. That's not a bad thing, but it's not a silver bullet either—just not yet, anyway. With each area having its own unique challenges, integrating technology into today's human condition is difficult. Every day the sun rises, we're still faced with a sea of sick and ill and unwell people who are in need of some form of guidance and assistance when it comes to health and well-being—human guidance and human assistance.

Good health starts outside the four walls of the clinical environment. It's nurtured and sustained in the home through human interaction between patient, family members, and other nonclinical support. Every patient journey is complex with a unique reality that cannot yet be captured with the use of a single app or other digital system. Apps might be valuable for tracking, guidance, and data collection, but the competency of the human using the tech is a crucial and complicated component.

Technology is incapable of looking someone in the face and understanding their point of view. It cannot have an in-depth conversation with a patient about their health beliefs and behaviors, or discuss with a caregiver what emotionally or economically compels a patient to adhere to behaviors that can help them. Apps will not soon be able to discuss the benefits and risks of an experimental treatment program with a patient or physician, or examine a community's cultural nuances with a clinical caregiver. Conversations are human exchanges of facts and emotions, empathy and insight, words and gestures. The human condition is dense, and no amount of artificial intelligence known to us today can replace the richness of nuance in human interaction.

Many in healthcare believe they'll derive solutions to complex challenges from an app or a novel user tech interface, and that better patient outcomes will result from these digital interactions—I think that's a risky assumption. The path of technology dependence that we're following in healthcare is on questionable ground. Are we overinvesting in technology and digital strategies while overlooking the richness of the patient's story and the nature of human interface? I think so. No amount of data or technology will ever replace human contact and understanding.

AI: AN INCOMPLETE SOLUTION?

In November of 2019, the Cambridge Union at Cambridge

University debated artificial intelligence (AI) and its value to humanity. To say the least, it was compelling. IBM Research's Project Debater, the first artificial intelligence platform capable of debating humans on complex topics, was the leading "speaker" on both the proposition and opposition. And the bottom line is important.

In an article published in the *Cambridge Independent* (the weekly newspaper for Cambridge University), the author, Adrian Peel, reported, "It was almost a little unnerving to hear that 'AI will not be able to make morally correct decisions, which can lead to disasters. It can only make decisions that it has been programmed to solve, whereas humans can be programmed for all scenarios.'" The bottom-line perspective of the debate was that "artificial intelligence will bring more harm than good." An interesting conclusion that is very serious, particularly in healthcare.

Another important point to consider when contemplating AI is IBM's own admission when they introduced Watson. Watson is the supercomputer that's the foundation for IBM's natural language processing platform. IBM clearly stated that Watson is probabilistic, not deterministic—meaning that it presented probabilities and did not determine anything. In healthcare, we have to understand, evaluate, and *determine* treatment paths using human beings. That little fact may never change.

Our use of technology in healthcare, and more specifically, our use of technology to support our human-centered marketing strategies in healthcare, is not negative—but our reliance on tech is naive. Unfortunately, instead of focusing on the patient's story, we've focused on how we can make technology work for us. As marketers, we should be employing methods to interact with patients and provide education and value at scale—methods that have a truly meaningful impact on the economics of healthcare. But instead, we've looked for an attractive shortcut—one that we've funded with both our money, and our time.

I'm not saying tech doesn't have a place in healthcare—clearly there are tech applications out there that look promising. But how do we assimilate apps and technology-based patient interfaces at scale and across a wide swath of patient types? It's not as easy as you might imagine—the human condition prevails. This is the challenge. I'm a proponent of human interaction whenever possible, but I've seen an app or two that I personally feel are great uses of technology in empowering patient or consumer competency.

Headspace, a company focused on helping people engage in mindfulness through technology, is what I would consider a good example of a health tech company seamlessly integrating a technology-driven interface into a patient-centric care delivery model. The mission of Headspace is to improve the health and happiness of the world—a big objective for a simple app. Users learn to meditate, and the foundational promise is one that, in my opinion, is grounded in behavioral health—and we all know how complicated the behavioral health space is.

Headspace stands out among health apps because the technology interacts with people by connecting them with a narrator—Andy Puddicombe, one of the founders—who guides users through the mindfulness journey. He instructs listeners on the principles of mindfulness, and how to open both their hearts and minds to the world around them in a way that makes them healthier and happier.

With one million subscribers and thirty-one million downloads, Headspace created a technological solution that empowers users to make lasting lifestyle changes—actually empowering them in their own health and well-being. People interact with the technology, using it to guide their behavior, rather than remember to take a pill or enter their weight. Many employers offer Headspace as a paid benefit for their employees. According to Headspace, the Headspace app had more than 250 corporate customers in 2019, and they anticipate this count to grow in future years. Companies like Google, Delta, and Roche offer Headspace as part of their benefits package, recognizing the growing acceptance of a multidimensional perspective of health and well-being.

The app has demonstrated that people can play an active role in their own health and well-being and that it's possible for technology to empower consumers to be competent patients. Not a bad thing, knowing that behavioral health problems such as anxiety and depression are largely present in the reality of many patients.

WHAT'S YOUR INTENTION?

As marketers, we search for smart ways to use our resources. *Our* intention is to use technology *and* traditional modes of marketing to support our brands and deliver our messages to the patient. We want our clients to reach their goals, whether that means more patients taking accountability for their health, increased filled prescriptions, or improved treatment plans. We want more personal interactions and fewer customers turning only to technology for their solutions. We want the patient to be at the heart of healthcare—which is exactly as it should be. And understanding their story and their point of view should be our first priority.

A rebirth in healthcare is coming, and through our efforts with ethnography and design thinking, we can be at the forefront of that change. It's not technology that's ushering in this rebirth—it's empathy and a willingness to put the patient at the center of it all.

CONCLUSION

No circle of influence is too small to make a difference in healthcare. You may not be a hospital CEO or administrator, or an agency principal, or the top executive at a pharmaceutical company—but that doesn't matter. Anyone in the healthcare system has the power to adopt a new mindset and shape the world around them.

In healthcare, we are the marketing, strategy, research, and innovation executives, and we share a particular advantage in this healthcare revolution. We are the communicators and the educators. We are the members of the healthcare community with the ability to engage with, educate, and empower patients *and* new ideas—and we can surely incite change. If we choose to embrace patient centricity, empathy is our best tool and biggest asset—we are champions of this rebirth. It starts with the patient, and we are their advocate.

If you've made it this far in reading this book, you're serious about championing a fresh perspective. You understand the role of empathy and human-centered approaches as a healthcare professional. As you go about the business of your career, you're ready to champion the tools of anthropology and design—especially when you think of patient education, competency, and accountability. With what you've learned here, you're ready to create brands that are relatable and accessible to patients so that fewer obstacles stand in their way on their journey towards competency.

I trust you feel motivated to become a champion for anthropology and design thinking, and that you seek to learn more about these powerful tools. You don't need a fancy degree to put the patient first, and you don't need an impressive title to use empathy as your guiding principle. In healthcare, we can always ask a patient to tell us their story. Why are they finding treatment difficult? Who helps them out of bed in the morning?

As long as we know where to start—and who to start with—we can use ethnography and design thinking in healthcare. Those marketing professionals who dig in and really seek to understand the patient reality and then leverage that understanding to the benefit of their brands will reap tremendous benefits.

It's important we start with the patient, but also remember the other stakeholders. Everyone has different insight and a multistakeholder approach is foundational to design. Only when we learn to collaborate amongst the multitude of stakeholders embedded in the business of healthcare, no matter their title, will we find the right solution. In patient centricity, the caregiver is equally as valuable as the patient. The perspective and trust of family members and patient advocates outside the clinical environment is paramount in our community. Working with both the patient and the caregiver, we're able to see the whole picture.

Understanding the patient experience may likely be the greatest innovation that has come to healthcare. We must continue the work of the innovators and make H2H healthcare the majority mindset. Champion the work of the anthropologist. Engage in design and learn how to become a design thinker. Become someone who changes the system. Working together—with the patient and his or her related stakeholders at the center of it all—we can make the healthcare world a better place for all of us.

SUGGESTED READING

Here are a few books you might be interested in reading:

- Kleinman, Arthur. *The Illness Narratives*. University of Michigan: Basic Books, 1988.
- Rogers, Everett M. *Diffusion of Innovations*. 5th ed. New York: Free Press, 2003.
- MacKenzie, Gordon. *Orbiting the Giant Hairball: A Corporate Fool's Guide to Surviving with Grace*. New York: Viking, 1998.
- Ku, Bon and Lupton, Ellen. *Health Design Thinking: Creating Products and Services for Better Health*. Massachusetts: The MIT Press, 2020.
- Guest, Kenneth J. *Essentials of Cultural Anthropology: A Toolkit for a Global Age*. 2nd ed. New York: W.W. Norton & Company, 2017.

And here is an interesting article:

- Fry, Erika and Schulte, Fred. "Death by a Thousand Clicks: Where Electronic Health Records Went Wrong." *Fortune*, March 18, 2019. https://fortune.com/longform/medical-records/

ACKNOWLEDGMENTS

Dave Chlastosz, Matt Bradley, and Diane McDonald for your selfless contributions in reading and guiding me as I crafted the narrative and manuscript.

Brian Shakley and the LIFT design team for helping me research and fact-check the manuscript, and for the illustrations in the book—you guys are amazing, and I am inspired by you all each and every day. Thank you for championing the vision.

Chris Snell for gently helping me see how valuable design and anthropology are in brand and marketing strategies.

J. Kevin Tugman for nudging me to get involved in the Mayo Clinic Center for Innovation and for pointing out the bedrock of LIFT.

All of our clients and partners at LIFT. You have given us the space to share our enthusiasm and provided us with the opportunity to prove the value of our vision.

ABOUT THE AUTHOR

DAVID MCDONALD is a founding partner and CEO of LIFT, a healthcare design and marketing firm devoted to the unique cause of patient-centered communication and experience design. LIFT specializes in human-centered insights and strategy for marketers seeking to impact Share of Experience®. LIFT is particularly attuned to the needs of hospitals/health systems and late-stage (phase 3 and post-regulatory) pharmaceutical company brands.

As a healthcare entrepreneur and anthropologist, David has worked for more than 25 years to advance the cause of patient education and well-being. David is passionate about human engagement and consumer behavior and is a thought leader in the life sciences for his use of ethnography and design thinking as tools to improve patient understanding and education. He is also the founder and current chair of The Institute for Healthcare Design Thinking.

David resides in Jupiter, Florida, with his wife Diane, and a dog called Oliver.